UNWANTED HAIR

Its cause and treatment

Ancestral Curse or Glandular Disorder?

UNWANTED HAIR
Its cause and treatment
Ancestral Curse or Glandular Disorder?

EDITED BY

Robert B. Greenblatt, M.D., C.M. (McGill)
Docteur Honoris Causa (Bordeaux)

Virendra B. Mahesh, Ph.D. (Delhi)
D.Phil. (Oxford)

R. Don Gambrell, Jr., M.D.
Diplomate, American Board of Obstetrics and Gynecology and Reproductive
Endocrinology

Medical College of Georgia
Augusta, Georgia

The Parthenon Press

Published by
The Parthenon Press
Casterton Hall
Carnforth, Lancs LA6 2LA
U.K.

ISBN 1-85070-103-2

Printed in the USA

DEDICATION

To Rose Mineni

For her devotion and tireless efforts to raise the standards in the treatment of the hirsute woman.

OTHER BOOKS BY THE AUTHORS
PERTAINING TO UNWANTED HAIR

THE HIRSUTE FEMALE, edited by Robert B. Greenblatt, M.D., Charles C. Thomas, Springfield, IL, 1963

HIRSUTISM AND VIRILISM, edited by Virendra B. Mahesh, Ph.D., D.Phil, and Robert B. Greenblatt, M.D., John Wright PSG Inc, Boston, Bristol, London, 1983

Grateful acknowledgement is due to the publishers, John Wright PSG, for permission to reproduce some of the material from the book *Hirsutism and Virilism*, edited by V. B. Mahesh and R. B. Greenblatt, 1983.

Contents

Contributors

Alice Berning, ED.D., R.E.
Assistant Professor Northern Illinois
University (Ret)
Assoc. Mary College
RR2 Box 275
Bismark, N.D. 58501

Norbert J. Berning, ED.D.
Assistant V.P. Mary College
RR2 Box 275
Bismark, N.D. 58501

Wendy Cooper
9 Applegrove, Reynoldston
Gower, SA3 1BZ, WALES

Karin H. Fischer
405 Ransdell Drive
Spartanburg, SC   29302

R. Don Gambrell, JR., M.D.
Clinical Professor of Endocrinology
and Obstetrics and Gynecology
Medical College of Georgia
Augusta, GA   30912

Robert B. Greenblatt, M.D.
Professor Emeritus of Endocrinology
Medical College of Georgia
Augusta, GA   30912

Ann L. Hyatt
Greenblatt & Gambrell Clinic
903 15th Street
Augusta, GA   30910

Anthony E. Karpas, M.D.
Internal Medicine Group Atlanta
478 Peachtree St., NE, Suite 207-A
Atlanta, GA   30308

Virendra B. Mahesh, PH.D., D. PHIL.
Regents Professor, Robert B. Greenblatt Professor
Chairman, Department of Endocrinology
Director, Center for Population Studies
Medical College of Georgia
Augusta, GA   30912

Paul G. McDonough, M.D.
Professor of Obstetrics and Gynecology
Director, Reproductive Endocrine Section
Medical College of Georgia
Augusta, GA   30912

Rose Mineni
Professional Electrolyis Continuing Education
Program
7709 McHenry Avenue
Modesto, CA   95356

Puthugramam K. Natrajan, M.D.
Assistant Professor of Endocrinology
and Obstetrics and Gynecology
Medical College of Georgia
Augusta, GA   30912

Santiago L. Padilla, M.D.
Assistant Professor of Obstetrics and
Gynecology
Reproductive Endocrine Section
Medical College of Georgia
Augusta, GA   30912

Foreword

Virendra B. Mahesh, Ph.D., D.Phil.

The growth and distribution of hair on the head and face of men and women has been a subject of much attention as well as concern over the ages. There are at least two reasons for the high degree of emphasis on head and facial hair. The growth of facial hair and the distribution of head hair in a man has been associated with his masculinity. Unwanted facial hair and/or recession of the hairline of the head has likewise been associated with the lack of feminity in women. In addition, the high emphasis on physical appearance in recent years has resulted in men seeking relief from baldness and women seeking relief from unwanted facial hair with vigor.

In the women's quest for the absence of facial hair both for the purpose of physical appearance as well as an expression of her femininity, it sometimes becomes difficult to judge whether the facial hair of the patient is within the realm of normal variation or excessive. This statement pertains only to those cases when there is a difference of opinion between the patient and the physician whether excessive facial hair is present or not. The confusion exists because there is no rigid or standard criterion as to what constitutes excessive facial hair growth to distinguish a borderline case from a normal case. Defining the pattern of normal hair distribution is further complicated by the wide variations in hair growth based on racial factors. As an example, Mongolians grow less body and facial hair as compared to Caucasians. A physiological basis of this difference in hair distribution is not currently known.

The growth of sexual hair is regulated by a class of steroid hormones called androgens. Often this class of hormones is referred to as the "male sex hormone" which is not scientifically correct. A variety of androgenic compounds are secreted by the adrenal gland, testes, and the ovaries in normal men and women. These compounds may have weak or strong androgenic activity, depending upon their structure. In the ovaries, these compounds are the precursors from which estrogens, the so called "female sex hormones", are synthesized. The term, "female sex hormones", for estrogens is as much a misnomer as the term, "male sex hormones", for androgens because estrogens are also synthesized and secreted in the normal male. The main difference in the male and female secretory patterns of hormones that influences sexual hair growth and sexual function is therefore not the type of hormones secreted but the quantity of the androgen, testosterone, and the estrogen estradiol secreted.

Across races such as Mongolians versus Caucasians, it is difficult to explain the differences in the distribution of sexual hair based on the levels of circulating androgens in blood due to limitations of our current knowledge in the regulation of hair growth. However, within the same race, the growth of excessive sexual hair is related to the level of biologically active androgens. These excessive androgens may be present, due to either their administration to the patient in form of drugs or abnormal functions of the adrenal and/or the ovaries or alterations in the metabolism of androgens. Excessive androgens may be produced by the adrenal and/or the ovaries, either by minor shifts in the ratio of androgens of high biological activity to those with lower biological activity, or minor shifts in the ratio of androgens to estrogens or by production of large quantities of the hormone due to stress-effects, hyperplasia or the presence of a tumor. Excessive androgen formation by the adrenals or the ovaries may not exclusively be the cause of hirsutism. Weak androgens, such as dehydroepiandrosterone, can be converted to the potent androgen, testosterone, in organs such as the liver. The differences in the extent of such conversion from individual to individual may very well relate to differences in the pattern of hair growth. Such differences may also be manifested in the metabolic breakdown products of testosterone to biologically-active and biologically-inactive metabolites. Furthermore, testosterone circulates in the blood stream in the form of the free unbound hormone and as the hormone bound to a blood protein. It is the free unbound hormone that manifests biological activity and the extent of protein binding thus dictates how much biological activity a certain amount of circulating testosterone can exert. Finally, testosterone is converted to a metabolic dihydrotestosterone before it acts on the hair follicle. The amount of enzyme present for this conversion in the hair follicle itself may determine the rate of its growth in response to androgens.

The above discussion points to the complexity of the question in trying to find an answer to the question as to the source of disorder in a particular woman causing excessive hair growth. With the progress of knowledge about the secretion and metabolism of androgens leading to improved methods of testing for the source of disorder, the androgen-producing disorder can be identified and treated in a large number of women. However, in spite of impressive advances made in the last two decades in methods of diagnosis of cause of hirsutism, there remains a large number of women with hirsutism in whom the cause of hirsutism cannot be determined. It is hoped that with further investigation in the cause of hirsutism which is being pursued vigorously throughout the world, better answers will be available in the future. The question remains as to what a woman with hirsutism and what her physician can do when the source of disorder cannot be discovered. Obviously, further diagnostic testing will not provide the answer until new methods are discovered that overcome the limitations of the current methods. The current method of management unfortunately lies in a trial and error approach by suppressing adrenal and/or ovarian function to reduce the level of circulating androgens to slow down the rate of hair growth along with the use of depilatories and electrolysis for the removal of hair. Antiandrogens are used extensively in Europe but the currently used European drug, Cyproterone Acetate, is not approved for use in the United States at the present time. Two new drugs of this type have been introduced in the United States however during the last three years.

This book provides an appraisal of what is currently known about the regulation of hair growth, the various causes of excessive androgen secretion, the current methods of diagnosis of the source of androgen excess and the current methods of management of hirsutism. Since the pathways of androgen biosynthesis are closely related in the adrenal, the ovaries and testes differing predominantly only in the mechanisms that control their secretion, certain segments of the presentation may appear repetitive but such repetition is necessary for the full presentation of the main topic under discussion.

Preface

Robert B. Greenblatt, M.D.

The removal of unwanted hair by electrolysis has reached a stage in development which makes the art a felicitous extension of the physician's regimen of treatment. Unwanted hair, especially facial, is a source of mental turmoil that often raises havoc with a woman's physiologic processes and her emotional stability. By far the greatest number of cases are idiopathic in origin, i.e., the result of a genetic (heritable) sensitivity of the hair follicle apparatus to one's normal levels of endogenous androgens (testosterone, etc.) or to a slight increase in production of these so-called male sex hormones by the ovaries and/or adrenals. It should be kept in mind that all sexual hair (face, axillary, pubis, abdomen, chest, etc.) is maintained by the so-called male sex hormones, although women normally produce these but in much smaller quantities than the male. Women suspected of suffering from an endocrinopathy, i.e., amenorrhea (absence of menstruation) and hirsutism or masculinizing symptoms such as voice changes, increase in muscle mass, enlargement of the clitoris, marked hairiness and receding hair line, require expert medical advice before undertaking electrolysis.

Much may be done to obtain a cosmetic result: (1) the administration of large doses of an estrogen along with cyclic courses of a progestin to attempt to suppress androgen production by the ovary and to increase the globulin in the blood that binds testosterone, thus lowering the availability of the 'free active testosterone' necessary for stimulation of the hair follicle apparatus. (2) Small doses of a corticoid such as prednisone or dexamethasone to partially suppress androgen secretion by the adrenals (for the severe cases). (3) Anti-androgen drugs such as spironolactone (Aldactone) or cimetidine (Tagamet). (4) Most importantly, to administer the coup de grace to the follicle producing the unwanted hair, i.e., destroying the hair follicle producing the unwanted hair by someone properly trained in the art and science of electrolysis.

The medical approach reduces the rate of sexual hair growth, prolongs the dormant period and delays the cyclicity. The physician can change the 'soil' favourable to hair growth, but the electrologist can eliminate the 'weeds'.

1
Electrolysis: The State of the Art

Norbert J. Berning, Ed.D.
Alice B. Berning, Ed.D.
Rose Mineni, R.E.

Queen Cleopatra, it is rumored, had a problem with unwanted hair. Whatever truth there is to the rumor, there is evidence that removal of unwanted hair dates to early times. In ancient Egyptian tombs, there are remains of abrasives that were probably used for the purpose. Because unwanted hair is a personal problem, there is nothing in history books that deals with it at any length. Even medical literature lacks extensive treatment of the matter. Until recently, doctors were too preoccupied with the more dramatic anatomical and physiological medical developments to get involved in a problem that is primarily social and psychologically personal.

Curiously, it was a St. Louis, Missouri oculist in the mid-nineteenth century who laid the groundwork for effectively eliminating unwanted hair. His work was prompted purely for medical reasons. Dr. Charles E. Michel had patients with hair growth abnormalities known as trichiasis (inverted eyelashes). Routinely, some sort of surgery and tweezing were the common solutions. The former, while successful, left scars and disfigured eyelids. Tweezing proved to be only a temporary remedy and actually caused the number of hairs in the area to increase and coarsen, thus making the problem even worse. However, Dr. Michel sought a way to remove the irritating hairs in a less formidable way.

Because he was well acquainted with the structure of the hair follicle, Dr. Michel concluded that destruction of the hair root and papilla would eliminate the hair growth. Somehow he had to get to the root, nourished by the papilla, and render it inactive. He was not a stranger to electricity and the effect it has on the skin structure. He reasoned that a slight charge into the follicle would bring about the desired change without causing harm to the patient. This theory led him to seek a source of electrical current that would be simultaneously safe and effective. He settled on the use of a battery. To this battery he connected a fine wire that could be inserted into the hair follicle leading to the papilla. His experiments with this technique not only proved successful, but marked the beginning of what is now known as electrolysis.

Dr. William A. Hardaway, a friend of Dr. Michel, was so inspired by this technique of removing hair that he adopted and expanded electrolysis in his work as a dermatologist. It is largely Dr. Hardaway's work that accounts for the development of present day electrolysis.

Electrolysis is the process of removing hair permanently by destroying the hair growing cells (papilla) with an electric current. Access to the papilla is made by inserting a very fine instrument into the hair follicle (Fig. 1). Through this fine instrument is transmitted a regulated and controlled electrical current from a highly sophisticated machine known as an epilator. The electric current cauterizes the papilla, thus rendering it impossible to produce more hairs. The process is performed by a highly trained professional called an electrologist.

Currently there are three types of electrolysis treatments that have been recognized by the American Medical Association as indisputably effective in permanent hair removal. One type is called galvanic, a direct current process that produces an electro-chemical formation of sodium hydroxide. This process congeals the papilla cells. A second type, thermolysis, uses indirect current that cauterizes the papilla, thus destroying the matrix with heat. Thermolysis is the most common type used in permanent hair removal because of its efficiency and speed. The third type of hair removal is called the super-imposed, a combination of galvanic and thermolysis.

There are other advertised types of hair removal that are not recognized as electrolysis. Some are various forms of do-it-yourself methods marketed through department stores and mail order catalogs. Some beauty salons now advertise a method known as electric tweezers, a technique being investigated by courts in several states as being fraudulent in claiming permanent hair removal. Other promoted devices include depilatory creams, waxing, pumice stones, shaving and tweezing. These are not only temporary expediencies but may result in an increased and coarser hair growth, and can cause rashes, blemishes, and even scarring.

Among the concerns women have when considering electrolysis treatments are the length of treatments, the pain factors involved during treatment and the number of treatments required for permanent removal of hairs from a particular part of the body.

There is no standard length of time for treatments that is suited to all individuals. Depending on a variety of conditions, the electrologist and client work out a treatment program. Generally, however, individual treatments last from fifteen minutes to one hour.

Individual reaction to the electrical impulse generated for hair removal differs. Some describe the sensation as a tingling feeling, a few report a warm reaction, and still others used the word 'pain' to describe it. Whatever the description, there are varying degrees of sensations that clients feel. Because of the nature of electrolysis there is bound to be some feeling when hairs are epilated. Hair, rooted in the dermal layer of the skin, is surrounded by a variety of nerve endings. Any disturbance to this anatomical structure is bound to cause a discomforting sensation. Additional conditions that can influence pain and its threshold are physiological variations caused by such factors as premenstrual stress, edema, lack of sleep, and family problems. Not infrequently, the client's fear (anticipated) of pain is greater than the actual (realized) sensation. A good electrologist is aware of these factors and conditions of the client's apprehension and therefore adjusts the treatment to the client's disposition.

Electrolysis is not a once only treatment remedy. One treatment might eliminate all the visible hairs, but because hair growth is not synchronized, there can be hundreds of hair follicles in the treated area which contain hairs either in the beginning growth stage or in a dormant state. Of the latter, some will spring into growth at unpredictable times, while others will never activate.

Perhaps the most important aspect of permanent hair removal is the normal hair growth cycle. All hairs go through a growth and replacement cycle, but these cycles are not consistent in length. However, common to each cycle are three stages (Fig. 2).

One stage is called anagen, the active growth period during which the hair grows, emerges through the skin surface, and matures. A second stage is known as catagen, the sloughing-off stage. These stages vary considerably with different hair areas. For example, head hairs usually remain active from two or four years before sloughing off, while eyebrows are shed in five to six months. A third stage, telogen or resting, is a time during which no hair is produced. The length of this stage is also not predictable nor consistent. In fact, some hairs are so virile that they do not go into a resting stage, while others might rest as long as a year or more. During the telogen stage the dermal papilla rebuilds its strength in preparation for the next hair to generate. It is estimated that 20% or more of the body's hair follicles are dormant at any given time.

Furthermore, hair growth cycles are not consistent in each individual, and factors such as age and physiological changes can affect the expression of each stage. Thus, for example, menopause activates facial hair growth in some women, whereas in others growth may slow down or cease entirely.

Additional factors which confront an electrologist in daily practice are the texture, moisture gradient, and hypo- or hyper-sensitivity of the skin; age

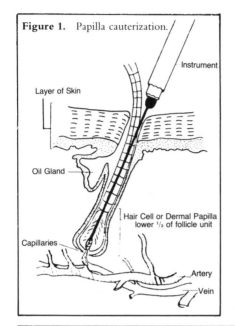

Figure 1. Papilla cauterization.

Instrument

Layer of Skin

Oil Gland

Hair Cell or Dermal Papilla lower ¹/₃ of follicle unit

Capillaries

Artery

Vein

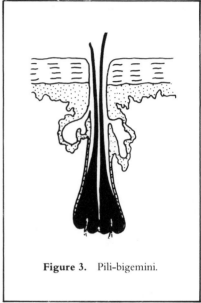

Figure 3. Pili-bigemini.

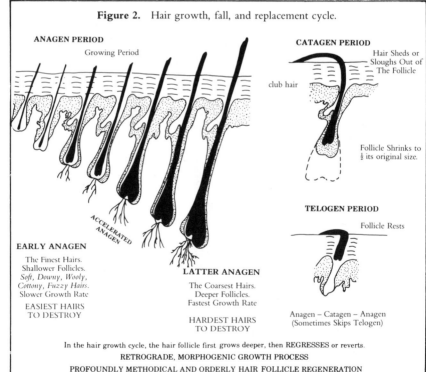

Figure 2. Hair growth, fall, and replacement cycle.

ANAGEN PERIOD

Growing Period

CATAGEN PERIOD

Hair Sheds or Sloughs Out of The Follicle

club hair

Follicle Shrinks to ½ its original size.

EARLY ANAGEN

The Finest Hairs.
Shallower Follicles.
*Soft, Downy, Wooly,
Cottony, Fuzzy Hairs.*
Slower Growth Rate

EASIEST HAIRS
TO DESTROY

ACCELERATED ANAGEN

LATTER ANAGEN

The Coarsest Hairs.
Deeper Follicles.
Fastest Growth Rate

HARDEST HAIRS
TO DESTROY

TELOGEN PERIOD

Follicle Rests

Anagen – Catagen – Anagen
(Sometimes Skips Telogen)

In the hair growth cycle, the hair follicle first grows deeper, then REGRESSES or reverts.

RETROGRADE, MORPHOGENIC GROWTH PROCESS

PROFOUNDLY METHODICAL AND ORDERLY HAIR FOLLICLE REGENERATION

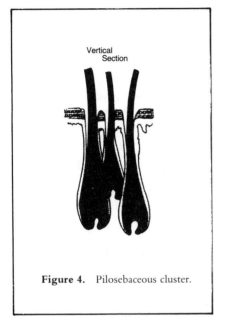

Vertical Section

Figure 4. Pilosebaceous cluster.

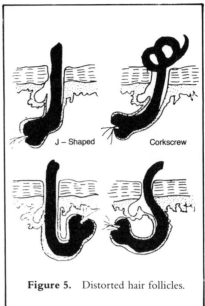

J – Shaped   Corkscrew

Figure 5. Distorted hair follicles.

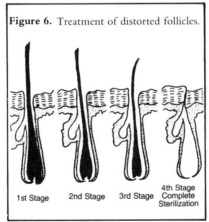

Figure 6. Treatment of distorted follicles.

1st Stage   2nd Stage   3rd Stage   4th Stage Complete Sterilization

and pain tolerance of the client; area of treatment; amount of previous tampering, e.g., tweezing, shaving, waxing; medication that may contribute to hair growth; stress; topical stimulation; skin grafts; surgical stimuli, etc.

Because of the growth cycle and other unique hair and skin characteristics, it can take from six months to a year or more to remove every hair from an area being treated. However, clients should realize that those who are faithful in taking treatments will find that the time for each treatment lessens as the time between treatments lengthens.

Multiple follicular hair units can also prolong the number of treatments. The units are of two kinds: two (pili-bigemini) or more (multi-gemini) hairs sharing one follicle (Fig. 3) and multi-follicular patterns which are two or more hairs (pilosebaceous clusters) in very close proximity (Fig. 4). Generally, these hairs are not simultaneously active. When the additional hairs in these units appear they give the impression of regrowth. Since these hairs are independent units they must be dealt with individually. Such hair units are most predominant in the upper thigh, panty line, lower leg, nipple, underarm and forearm areas.

In difficult cases, the first treatment may only partially destroy the hair matrix. Within a period ranging from five weeks to three months, the germ cell will reactivate and produce another hair, but it will be finer and less deep than the original. To prevent these finer hairs from rebuilding to their former strength, it is imperative to schedule treatments immediately after the new hairs appear.

Difficult cases are usually associated with hair follicles that are not straight. These occur in various forms — curved, twisted, 'U' or 'S' shaped (Fig. 5). Since the fine instrument used for electrolysis is straight, these curved (distorted) hairs will require several treatments to straighten the follicle, break it down, and finally cauterize the entire papilla effectively (Fig 6).

While coarse and deep hairs are found in the average woman, they are common in the woman with characteristics of masculine hirsutism. Such hirsutism is either inherited or developed by change in one's physiological conditions. The latter can be brought about by such factors as trauma, stress, ovarian disturbances, and other hormonal imbalances, medications, or by personal tampering through plucking, shaving, waxing, and depilatories.

In addition to permanent removal of hair, electrolysis provides other long-term permanent benefits. Accompanying the removal of unwanted hair is the elimination of an embarrassing physical appearance, the enhancement of self-image, and the resolution of a negative attitude. To many who are afflicted by unwanted hairs, these may seem frivolous and superficial benefits. Too frequently, however, it is only those who have endured the burden of unwanted hair who appreciate the value of such benefits. And it should be emphasized gently that often the most important people who do not understand the stresses caused by unwanted hair are the person's spouse and family, and even the family physician.

The physician, especially, is the natural target for counsel on this matter. Professionally he/she should exercise consideration and compassion when dealing with such a patient and at least suggest the only method of permanent hair removal recognized by the American Medical Association – electrolysis.

2
Hirsutism: Ancestral Curse or Endocrinopathy

Robert B. Greenblatt, M.D.

The clinician is apt to view every hairy female as an endocrine problem. In a larger sense, such a conclusion is essentially correct. When examined from the point of view that the hair follicle is an end-organ influenced and stimulated by certain hormones, then it would be fair to assume that 'all excessive hairiness' is indeed an endocrine problem, provided the roles of heredity, genetic factors, and sensitivity of the target gland receptors are considered.

Homo sapiens, in his phylogenetic development, emerged erect but void of the thick pelage which covers the bodies of all other primates. Neanderthal man, who lived in Europe some 70,000 to 40,000 years ago, lost some of the hairy tegument that covered the bodies of his earlier ancestors. The thick coarse hair of man's anthropid heritage remains only in a few areas, but the vestiges of this hair-covering persists as follicles producing fine, lightly pigmented lanugo (vellus) hair over most of the body's surface. The human remains potentially a naked ape and retains the capacity to grow coarse, thick terminal hair on face, chest, abdomen, back, extremities, along with pubic and axillary hair. Thus, human hair is of two types: vellus and terminal. Both types are found on all skin areas except the palms of the hand and soles of the feet, which have no hair follicles.[1]

The growth of hair is cyclic. There are three phases: anagen is the growing phase; catagen, the transitional period of rapid involution; telogen, the quiescent phase.[2] The duration and variation in anagen and telogen phases in the human depends on many factors, and unlike the hair follicles of animals which molt periodically, human hair follicles are not synchronized. Each follicle is supplied by one or more sebaceous glands which produce oil or sebum to lubricate the hair. In humans, excessive hairiness is usually accompanied by increased oiliness. To each hair follicle a special muscle is attached, the arrector pili. Downy vellus hair lacks this muscle. Human hair, as in some animals, can become erect in moments of great stress because of this special muscle. Shakespeare made this point quite explicit when the ghost of Hamlet's father said:

> I could a tale unfold whose lightest word
>   would harrow up thy soul;
> And each particular hair to stand on end.

Hair is second only to skin as a physical sign of racial difference. Almost all Mongolians (Chinese, Japanese, Koreans, American Indians, Eskimos) have dark straight coarse hair on their heads; it is crinkly or wooly in the Negro, and curly or straight in the Caucasian. As for body and facial hair, the Mongolian, Negroid and American Indian races are noticeably less hirsute than Caucasians, and among the Caucasians, there are ethnic differences: hair growth is heavier in those of Mediterranean than in those of Nordic ancestry.

Man's interest and fascination with hair – absence or excess – have been known since recorded time. The Bible relates that Esau's body and arms were covered by an abundance of hair; Aristotle wondered why eunuchs failed to grow beards but maintained their full head of hair; St. Paul wrote that a woman's head hair is "her crowning glory". In all generations however, the bearded woman has been the object of great curiosity, and the subject of much derision. The storied legends of the past have designated the bearded woman as an unnatural individual. Shakespeare seized upon this motif when he wrote about the three weird sisters in *Macbeth:*

> You should be women and yet
>   Your beards forbid me
> To interpret that you are so.

The statue of a bearded lady stands in Westminster Abbey. She is Saint Wilgefort, a Portugese princess who was betrothed against her will to a suitor she did not love. According to legend, she prayed that she might become so unattractive that he would no longer wish to marry her. Her prayers were answered – she grew a coarse beard which repelled her suitor. Saint Wilgefort then devoted the rest of her life to religion and died a virgin.[3] Does such a case purport to underline a possible influence of the psyche as a factor in abnormal sexual hair growth? Indeed, hirsutism is said to be far more prevalent in women confined to institutions for the insane. Bush and Mahesh reported a temporary increase in facial hairiness in a woman following an ill-fated love affair. The abnormal hairiness regressed soon after a favorable resolution of the situation. They were able to demonstrate an increased production of adrenal androgens during the period of emotional stress.[4]

Quite a different message issues from the celebrated painting "La Barbuda" by Jusepe de Ribera which hangs in the Tavera Hospital Museum in Toledo, Spain. In 1631, Ribera portrayed a 52-year-old woman from Naples with a luxuriant beard nursing her infant, and her somewhat meek husband standing beside her (Fig. 1). At age 37, after she had experienced three spontaneous abortions, the growth of facial hair began. The reproductive history of this woman suggests some hormonal disturbance for the unusual course of events. Ribera, much against his esthetic sense, was commissioned by the Duke of Alcala to record for posterity this unique phenomenon.[5]

The masculine distribution of hair in a girl or woman is not only a cosmetic catastrophy, but is also a source of considerable anguish and emotional trauma. Excessive growth of hair on the face of a woman, known as hirsutism, may or may not be accompanied by menstrual disorders or unwanted hair on the chest and abdomen. Although hirsutism is often regarded as presumptive evidence of a lack of femininity, it need not be a deterrant to essential womanhood or functional fertility.[6] However, when clitoral hypertrophy (enlargement), varying degrees of regression of the cephalic hair line or even male pattern baldness, deepening of the voice, increased muscle mass,

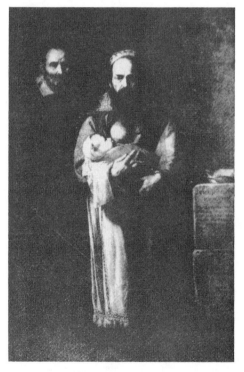

Figure 1.   The celebrated "La Barbuda" by Ribera, a 52-year-old bearded woman nursing her child, hangs in the Museum of the Tavera Hospital at Toledo, Spain. She became markedly hirsute at age 37 after having had three spontaneous abortions. The picture, commissioned by the Duke of Alcala, serves to place on record that hirsute women have become and do become mothers.

and amenorrhea (in almost all instances) are accompaniments of hirsutism, then the symptom-complex is called 'virilism.' On the other hand, hypertrichosis is a term frequently employed to denote overgrowth of hair on arms, thighs and legs, and sometimes of the back, which may or may not be associated with facial hirsutism or virilism.

FACTORS INFLUENCING THE GROWTH OF HAIR

Some knowledge of the biology of hair growth and its relationship to the endocrine system is essential for an understanding of aberrations in hair distribution. Hair is a derivative of the epidermis, and the hair follicle is a component of the pilosebaceous apparatus. The full complement of these units is present three months before birth, and it is unlikely that hair follicles can develop *de novo* in the human adult. There are no differences between the male and female in the distribution of hair follicles. The difference in sexual hair patterns between males and females is due mainly to the titer of circulating androgens. Thus, the tendency to abnormal hairiness in the female remains quiescent, but may burgeon forth at any time because of a variety of intrinsic and extrinsic factors (Table 1).

In the human, facial hair follicles, like those for pubic and axillary hair, lie more or less dormant until puberty, becoming fully active only under the chemical impulses of androgenic hormones. As has been mentioned already, aside from hormonal influences there are genetic or hereditary factors involved as well. The plasma concentration of testosterone in Japanese males and females is the same as in Caucasians.[7] However, there is a systemic difference in the sensitivity of the epidermal appendages to androgens; hirsutism is extremely rare in Japanese women, as is acne. Furthermore, Japanese women tolerate exogenous androgens in doses which result in hirsutism or even masculinization in Caucasian females.

In rats, estrogens retard the initiation and rate of hair growth and produce a finer hair; androgen induces a coarse pelage. Hormones, such as androgens and growth hormone, increase the rate of hair growth, while estrogens decrease the diameter of hair produced. Estrogens not only decrease the rate of anagen activity but also lessen sebum activity.

Table 1   Factors Influencing Abnormal Hairiness in the Female

1. An inborn androgen sensitivity of the pilosebaceous apparatus
2. Undue metabolic clearance rates of certain endogenous androgens
3. A decrease in testosterone's protein-binding capacity
4. An inherent facility for androgen conversion to testosterone and/or to dihydrotestosterone
5. Psychogenic stresses that either increase adrenal androgen output or modify pilary responsiveness
6. Endocrinopathies which produce increased amounts of androgens – seen in certain ovarian and adrenal disorders

All body processes are temperature sensitive and the skin is much more subject to changes in environmental temperature than any other organ. Hair growth in the human, as well as in a variety of mammals, is more rapid in the summer. Increased blood flow and the resultant increase in dermal temperature are probably responsible for increased local hair growth in areas chewed or sucked by psychotic patients, in areas overlying bone fractures, or unilaterally on the side of sympathectomy.[8]

ACTION OF ANDROGENS

Male and female epidermal teguments are quite similar, as is steroidogenesis for the adrenals, the ovaries and testes. Androgens derive from the adrenals, testes and ovaries. The ovary converts nonandrogenic C_{21} steroids (pregnenolone and progesterone) into androgenic steroids which then covert to estrogens. Androgens, whether of adrenal or gonadal origin, are the obligatory estrogen precursors. Estrogens are more efficiently produced in the female and these hormones are believed to limit testosterone's physiologic action by increasing its protein-binding capacity. However, derangements in the pathways for estrogen synthesis resulting in increased androgen turnover may readily occur. All these factors – and many more – are at play to create hirsutism and hypertrichosis.[9-14]

We can think of the skin as an enormous endocrine gland. It extracts androgens from the circulation, binds them and converts them to both more active and inactive products. Certain skin – the prepuce, for example – can convert androgens to dihydrotestosterone more readily than other tissues. It is dihydrotestosterone, derived from testosterone and perhaps in even greater amounts from ∇^4-androstenedione, which acts at the receptor – protein level in the hair-follicle cell. In instances where there is an inherent defect in the receptor sites — the feminizing insensitive androgen syndrome — neither testosterone nor dihydrotestosterone will induce hair growth, acne, clitoral hypertrophy or voice changes (Fig. 2). On the other hand, certain endocrine states play a permissive role for hairiness. The hypertrichosis of juvenile hypothyroidism and the hirsutism observed following large chronic doses of cortisone are not due to excessive androgens.

Many hirsute females do not manifest any obvious or latent disorder in endocrine balance. Secondary sexual characteristics such as bodily contour, breast development, fat depots, may be completely on the distaff side. The menstrual cycles may be regular and ovulatory, and the ability to conceive and bear children may not be impaired in any way. Her aptitudes and attitudes may remain astonishingly feminine; pelvic measurements usually reveal the perfect gynecoid pelvis and hormonal surveys may reveal normal serum androgen levels. Why then the hirsutism?

Excessive hair growth may be caused by an increased sensitivity of the hair

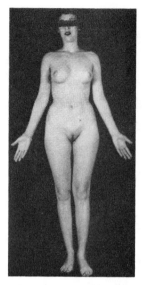

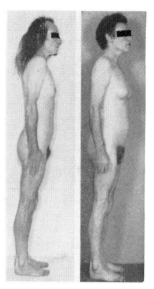

Figure 2. A 21-year-old woman with syndrome of feminizing abdominal testes. Note absence of all sexual hair. (Reproduced with permission from Greenblatt, R. B., Recent Prog Hor Res 14:335, 1958.)

Figure 3. A and B. Adrenal adenoma in a 41-year-old female. Note hypertrichosis of extremities and cephalic alopecia. Clitoris was slightly enlarged, facial hair growth was mild. (Reproduced with permission from Greenblatt, R. B., *The Hirsute Female,* Springfield, IL., Chas. C. Thomas, 1965.)

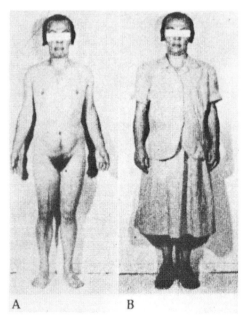

A   B

Figure 4. A and B. Long-standing congenital adrenal hyperplasia in a 32-year-old female. Note absence of breast development, male escutcheon, cephalic alopecia. Patient shaved daily.

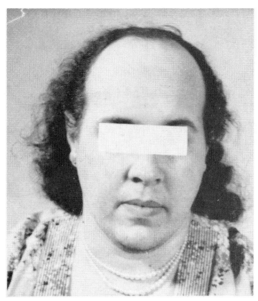

Figure 5. Hirsutism and cephalic alopecia in a woman 38 years old without any other signs or symptoms of masculinization; gravida IV, para II.

follicle to endogenous androgens. This may be either a dominant or a recessive hereditary trait. On the other hand, in the greater number of hirsute women with so-called idiopathic hirsutism, there may be minor to major enzymatic defects in the biosynthesis of certain steroids by the ovary or adrenal, or there may be disturbances in intrinsic liver or kidney metabolism which may alter the nature and rate of excretion of different steroids. According to Ishmail et al[15] and Vermeulen,[16] anomalies of androgen metabolism, however mild, can be demonstrated in a majority of women with so-called idiopathic hirsutism if sophisticated endocrine studies are performed. The question may then be asked, "Is hirsutism an ancestral curse or is it an endocrinopathy?"

All hair growth, wherever it is on the body, may be said to be hormone-dependent. However, it is the facial (beard) hair, axillary hair, chest hair, and the abdomino-pubic hair that is considered 'sexual hair'. Such hair growth is directly dependent on the glands of internal secretion and appears only after androgens, which were produced by the adrenals and gonads, have made their presence felt over a sufficient length of time. Although head hair is not considered primarily as sexual hair, nevertheless it cannot be said to be entirely a genetic feature for head hair and the hair line are markedly modified by gonadal and adrenal hormones. Baldness in men follows a genetic pattern, tempered by the individual hormonal milieu. Degrees of baldness are also seen in women without obvious endocrinopathies, while mild to marked cephalic alopecia may be seen in women harboring virilizing ovarian or adrenal tumors (Fig. 3 a,b), or women with long-standing congenital adrenal hyperplasia (Fig. 4 a,b), as well as in women without any other stigmata of masculinization (Fig. 5).

Men castrated in their youth may not ever become bald in spite of a familial history of baldness, and bald men have been known in occasional instances to regrow their hair following castration. Loss of head hair, eye lashes, eye brows and bodily hair, i.e., pubic hair and hair on the extremities, may occur after certain illnesses such as typhoid fever, and after ingestion of toxic drugs. Some auto-immune disorder which is often aggravated by deep emotional conflicts may be associated with alopecia universalis, loss of all hair on the head, eyebrows, eyelids, and on the body, and patchy loss of scalp hair (alopecia areata). It is of interest that pregnancy, stress of surgery, and other unexplained occurrences may temporarily restore bodily and head growth in cases of alopecia universalis and areata. Incidentally, chronic therapy with corticoids has been employed with considerable success in restoring hair growth in a large proportion of women with alopecia areata and in a lesser number of those with alopecia totalis (Fig. 6 a-d).

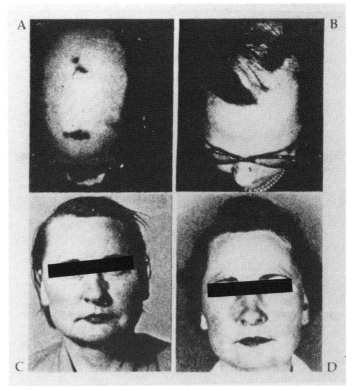

Figure 6. A – D. Alopecia areata – note excellent response to oral glucocorticoid therapy.

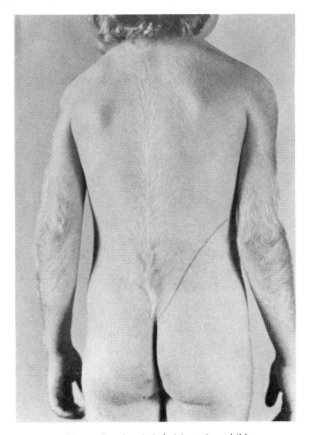

Figure 7.   Atavistic hairiness in a child.

Hairiness of the extremities more closely fits into a genetic pattern but is also influenced by endogenous and exogenous hormones. The hypertrichosis that is seen on the arms and backs of children (Fig. 7) is probably an atavistic manifestation and a throw-back to an ancestral form of body covering. Hypothyroidism has been incriminated in certain cases, but most of these children do not show evidence of hypothyroidism, nor do they respond to thyroid medication.

Hair that is present at birth and in infancy is said to be 'genetic;' that which appears after puberty is said to be 'sexual'. The response of the hair follicle apparatus depends on the state of nutrition, hereditary factors, and end-organ sensitivity. Young women suffering from anorexia nervosa (a disorder with psychogenic, nutritional and endocrine components) may exhibit a growth of fine lanugo hair on their bodies which at times may be quite marked (Fig. 8). Actually, the stimulus for sexual hair growth is an androgenic one in both male and female.[10] Estrogens, somatotropins, and thyroid hormone influence and modify but are not responsible, per se, for hair growth. In hypothyroid-ism, the growth of sexual hair is scanty and head hair may be dry and brittle. In hypocorticoidism (Addison's disease) sexual hair is decreased in the female and may be decreased in the Addisonian male if he also has poor testicular function. Large doses of corticoids, as first used by Hench for the manage-ment of rheumatoid arthritis, often induced unwanted hair growth, and so for a while the sobriquet of the 'hairy hormone' was applied to cortisone. Small doses have been used with a modicum of success in the management of those women thought to have hirsutism of adrenal origin, i.e., those with increased levels of dehydroepiandrosterone sulfate.[17] In hypopituitarism, sexual hair is, as a rule, quite scanty and pubic hair may be completely absent.

The major role of androgens and the negative role of estrogens in promot-ing pubic hair growth is strikingly demonstrated by young women with sexual infantilism due to primary pituitary failure. Estrogen and progestogen administration will induce breast growth and menstrual periods, but pubic and axillary hair will appear only after androgen administration. Note that pubic hair growth occurred only after androgens but not estrogens in a woman with hypopituitarism caused by a craniopharyngioma (Fig. 9 a–c).

For many years the adrenal was thought to be the sole source of androgens in the female, but the contribution of the ovary to the androgen pool is no longer in dispute. In certain instances, extirpation of the ovaries has been followed by marked regression of unwanted hair. Such a procedure in young women is, of course, out of the question, but in one case of hirsutism in a

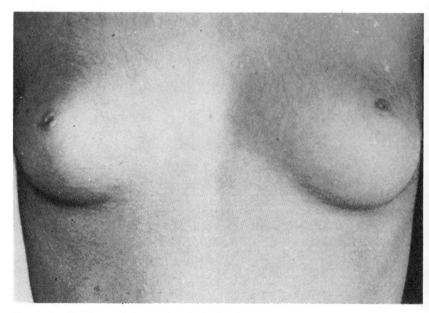

Figure 8.   Fine lanugo hair covering the body of a young woman with anorexia nervosa.

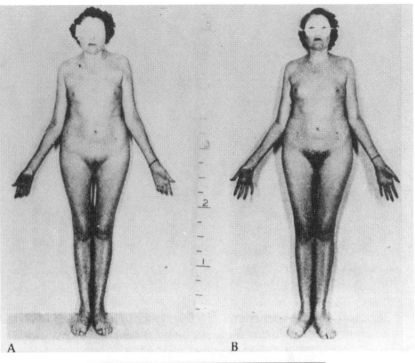

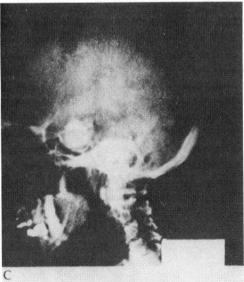

Figure 9.   A – C. Sexual infantilism in a woman with craniopharyngioma. Menses and breast development followed estrogen and progestogen therapy, but pubic hair growth occurred only after the addition of androgens to the hormonal regimen.

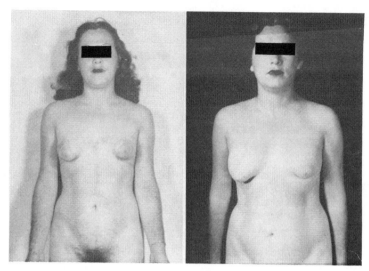

Figure 10. A and B. Definite regression of excess facial and bodily hair growth followed panhysterectomy in a young woman with acanthoma of the uterus.

woman aged 28 years with uterine bleeding resulting from an endometrial cancer, panhysterectomy was followed within a few months by regression of well over 80 percent of the unwanted hair growth (Fig. 10 a,b).

CONCLUSIONS

To better understand the complexity of abnormal hair growth, consideration must be given to genetic, psychogenic, and hormonal factors, as well as the inherent sensitivity of androgen receptors for sexual hair growth. The study of hair growth patterns in many of nature's experiments – alopecia areata and universalis, sexual infantilism, masculinizing adrenal tumors and congenital adrenal hyperplasia, ovarian neoplasms and dysfunctional ovarian and adrenal disorders – have provided insights into the many factors influencing growth of sexual hair. By far the greatest number of women with hirsutism have either an hereditary or genetic background or some subtle change in their androgen production and metabolism. It may be justifiable to say then that hirsutism is both an ancestral curse and an endocrinopathy.

References

1. Hamilton, J. B., Effect of castration in adolescent and young males upon further changes in the proportions of bare and hairy scalp. J. Clin Endocrinol Metab 20:1309, 1960
2. Ferriman, D., *Human Hair Growth in Health and Disease*. Kugelmass IN (ed). Springfield, IL, Charles C. Thomas, 1971
3. Cooper, W., *Hair: Sex, Society, Symbolism*. New York, Stein and Day Publishers, 1971, p 29
4. Bush, I. E., and Mahesh V. B., Adrenocortical hyperfunction with sudden onset of hirsutism. J. Endocrinol 18:1, 1959
5. Greenblatt, R. B., *The Hirsute Female*. Springfield, IL, Charles C. Thomas, 1965
6. Greenblatt, R. B. and Mahesh, V. B., Clinical evaluation and treatment of the hirsute female. In, *The Hirsute Female*. Clin Obstet Gynecol 7:1109, 1964
7. Kobayashi, T., Lobotsky, J. and Lloyd C. W., Plasma testosterone in urinary 17-ketosteroids in Japanese and Occidentals. J. Clin Endocrinol Metab 26:610, 1966
8. Segre, E. J., *Androgens, Virilization and the Hirsute Female*. Kugelmass IN (ed). Springfield, IL, Charles C. Thomas, 1967
9. Abraham, G. E., Chakmakjian Z. H., and Buster, J. E., et al: Ovarian and adrenal contributions to peripheral androgens in hirsute women. Obstet Gynecol 46:169, 1975
10. Mahesh, V. B., Greenblatt, R. B., and Aydar, C. K., et al: Urinary steroid excretion patterns in hirsutism. I. Use of ovarian and adrenal suppression tests in the study of hirsutism. J. Clin Endocrinol 23:1238, 1964
11. Kirschner, M. A., Bardin, C. W., and Hembree, W. C., et al: Effect of estrogen administration on androgen production and plasma luteinizing hormone in hirsute women. J. Clin Endocrinol 30:727, 1970
12. Gordon, G. G., Southern, A. L., and Tochimoto, S., et al: Effect of medroxyprogesterone acetate (Provera) on the metabolism and biological activity of testosterone. J. Clin Endocrinol 30:449, 1970
13. Odell, W. D., Ross, G. T., and Rayford, P. L., Radioimmunoassay for luteinizing hormone in human plasma or serum: Physiological studies. J. Clin Invest 46:248, 1967
14. Bardin, C. W., and Lipsett M. B., Testosterone and androstenedione blood production rates in normal women and women with idiopathic hirsutism or polycystic ovaries. J. Clin Invest 46:891, 1967
15. Ismail, A. A. A., Davidson, D. W., and Souka, A. R., et al: The evaluation of the role of androgens in hirsutism and the use of a new anti-androgen "Cyproterone acetate" for therapy. J. Clin Endocrinol Metab 29:81, 1974
16. Vermeulen, A., quoted by Hammerstein, J., Round-table Discussion. In *Androgenization in Women*. Hammerstein, J., Lachnit-Fixson, U., Neumann N., Plewig, G., (eds). Amsterdam, Excerpta Medica ICS 493, 1980, p 276
17. Greenblatt R. B., Cortisone in treatment of hirsute women. Am J Obstet Gynecol 66:700, 1953

3
The Anatomy of the Skin and Physiology of Hair Growth

Karin H. Fischer
Ann L. Hyatt

Why man evolved without the thick pelage that covered the bodies of his anthropoid ancestors, or why he retained vestiges of coarse hair growth only on certain areas of the body, are questions as old as mankind itself, and for which modern science still has no ready answers. However, it is known that man's lack of hairiness is not due to a lack of hairs, for in fact a chimpanzee is said to have fewer hair follicles on its body than does an adult human.[1] Hair follicles appear in every part of human skin except for the palms of the hands and soles of the feet, but most of man's hairs have become small, relatively colorless and unobtrusive. The pilosebaceous unit (the hair follicle together with its sebaceous glands) is a rudimentary skin appendage responsive to heredity, nutrition, and hormones.

Man's skin is not only the heaviest, and most visible organ, next to the brain it is one of the most complex. Within this outer covering, or integument, that is all too often taken for granted, are countless millions of intricate structures and mechanisms that connect the skin and its appendages to the entire organism of the human body. Connected to the brain via the central nervous system and to the other organs and endocrine system via the blood supply, the skin is an integral component of the body that provides a 'window' on the inner body to reflect the general state of the body's health.[2]

In the field of medicine, disorders of the skin and its appendages are normally assigned to the realm of the dermatologist; but because the skin and its appendages are hormone responsive or dependent, they also fall into the realm of the endocrinologist. Until recently the only contact between the two specialities was through personal 'friendships'.[3] Today, the two branches of medicine are collaborating to find solutions to the age old problem of unwanted hair which is so emotionally devastating to afflicted women. The electrologist must be added to this medical collaboration, because once hirsutism begins, though further development may be arrested and gradually reduced hormonally, the established hairs remain and continued growth can only be stopped by permanent removal. Therefore, for a better understanding of abnormal hair growth, this chapter will deal specifically with the anatomy and functions of the skin and its appendages, and the physiology of normal hair growth. Other chapters will define the causes of unwanted hair and cures.

ANATOMY AND FUNCTIONS OF THE SKIN AND APPENDAGES

The major function of the skin is protection. It is the largest of the body's organs of the senses, and is the physical barrier between man and the environment in which he lives. In an average adult, the skin measures about 2.0 m² in size (equal to a sheet 6 x 3 feet), accounts for approximately 15% of total body weight (equal to 22 pounds in a 150 pound adult), and varies in thickness over different areas of the body from a thirty-second to a tenth of an inch.[4,5] The skin must be very elastic to adapt to the nearly continuous movements of the body, and though it appears smooth over most of the body, in some areas it is thick, taut, rough and furrowed. In other areas it is thin, lax, and translucent. It contains multitudinous patterns of ridges, folds and whorls, which begin to develop in the thirteenth week of fetal life, and are distinct and different in each individual. Though the skin is incredibly alive and is constantly shedding dead cells and renewing itself, these distinct patterns do not change thoughout life and can only be altered by injury, scarring and calluses, or by deliberate surgical manipulation.

The skin provides the human body its first line of protection from invasion of noxious chemicals, lethal bacteria, fungi, parasites, and entrance of damaging amounts of ultraviolet irradiation. It also protects the inner body from injury by low-voltage electrical current, damage due to shocks or mechanical forces, extreme environmental temperatures, and prevents the loss of body fluids.

The skin's biochemical function is also of great importance to man. When exposed to sunlight, it has the ability to transform Vitamin D₂ (also called pro-Vitamin D) into Vitamin D₃, which is essential to human metabolism. A lack of Vitamin D leads to serious bone changes. From the blood stream it extracts and synthesizes endocrine hormones that produce and maintain hair growth. In the field of medicine, the skin has become a vital organ for vaccination to protect against a variety of diseases, such as smallpox, measles, mumps, diptheria and typhoid fever, and has now become invaluable in the field of allergy testing as well.

Layers of the skin

The skin is composed of three layers: (1) the epidermis (outer layer), (2) the dermis (corium or true skin), and (3) the panniculus adiposus (subcutaneous tissue). Below the subcutaneous tissue is a discontinuous flat sheet of skeletal muscle, the panniculus carnosus, which separates the skin from the rest of the body tissue. Figure 1 depicts a cross section of skin and its various structures. The appendages within are the sweat glands, hair follicles and sebaceous glands; each of these structures will be discussed separately (Fig. 2).

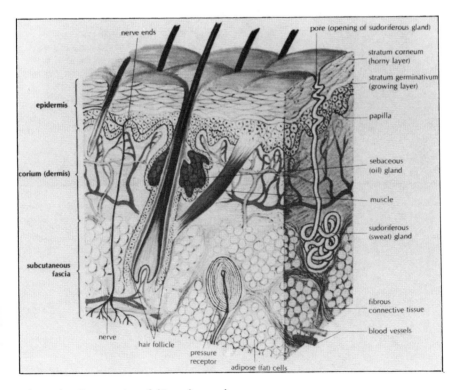

Figure 1.   Cross-section of skin and appendages.
(Courtesy of J. B. Lippincott Co., Philadelphia, from their publication *Structure and Function of the Human Body,* edited by Memmler Lundeen, R, Wood, D. L., 1977.)

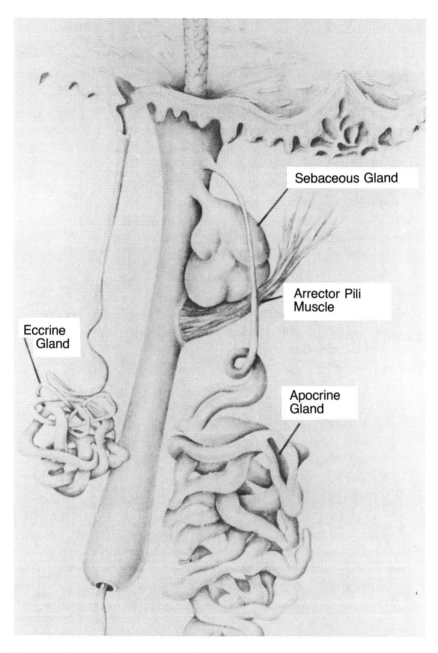

Figure 2. Diagram of cutaneous appendages.
(Courtesy of Montagna, W. and Parakkal, P. F., *The Structure and Function of Skin*. New York, Academic Press, 1974.)

The epidermis

The epidermis is non-vascular and consists of stratified epithelium (four or five layers of different cells). It has no blood supply of its own and is dependent on the vascular connective tissue bed (the dermis) below it for nourishment and removal of waste products. Describing the epidermis, Malphigi (circa 1669) divided it into an inner or basal layer of viable cells (called stratum Malphigi), and an outer one of anucleated horny cells. These two layers are subdivided into the following five strata, listed here from the deepest to the outermost layer:

1.   Stratum germinativum (germinating layer), consists of cuboidal or low columnar cells with the long axis oriented perpendicularly to the skin surface. As these cells divide and ascend toward the surface, they become larger and of different shape, and begin to synthesize a loose filamentous protein.

2.   The stratum spinosum (spiny layer of variable thickness) is composed of several layers of cells which become larger, polyhedral (many-sided) and, toward the granular layer above, progressively flatten and are oriented horizontally to the skin surface. The cells are connected by spindle-shaped cell junctions called 'desmosomes'.[6,7] This fibrous protein appears to be more compact.

3.   The stratum granulosum (granular layer) is composed of one or two rows of oval, horizontally oriented cells containing keratohyalin granules.

4.   The stratum lucidum (hyalin, clear layer). This thin clear layer of flattened, closely packed cells is present between the granular layer and stratum corneum only in areas of the body where the epidermis is very thick (as in the palms of the hands or soles of the feet) or in friction surfaces.

5.   The stratum corneum (outer, horny or cornified layer) is composed of highly organized units of horny, flattened cells, stacked in vertical columns one above the other. In friction surfaces, the cells of the thick horny layer are firmly cemented together.

As the epidermal cells migrate upward from the germinating layer, they lose most of their mitotic activity by differentiating into filaments, membrane coating granules, keratohyalin, and thickened plasma membrane and finally become constituents of the horny outer layer. The keratinized cells of the horny layer are dead cells and are continuously shed and replaced by cells from the germinative layer, which receives most of the diffused nutrients from the connective tissue of the dermis that lies immediately below.

Pigment granules responsible for skin color are manufactured by melanocytes in the basal layer (stratum germinativum). Melanocytes transfer pigment granules to the adjoining epidermal cells. In individuals with light colored skin, the pigment is limited to the basal layer; in dark-skinned races, melanin is found throughout the germinating and granular layers. A sun-tan and/or freckles are due to proliferation of these granules under the stimulus of sunlight.

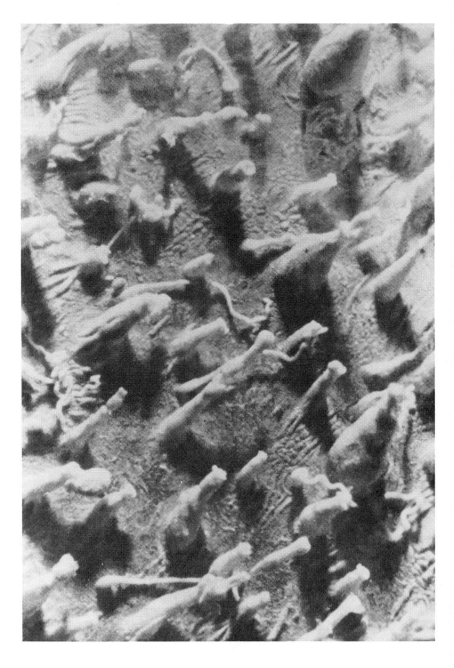

Figure 3. The underside of the epidermis of an eyelid showing many small hair follicles and the relatively flat dermo-epidermal junction, except at the base of the hair follicle. (From: IBID)

The distinctive features of the human epidermis are a relatively high total thickness and a well developed dermo-epidermal function. Its thickness varies from 0.07 to 1.4 mm; it is thinnest in the eyelids and thickest in the soles of the feet (plantar skin) and palms of the hands (palmar skin).[8] The understructure of the epidermis is variable, irregular, with cones, ridges and cords of diverse lengths extending at different depths into the dermis. Through this uneven terrain, usually at the tip of the ridges, the ducts of the sweat glands and pilary canals of the hair follicle enter. Hair follicles and the sebaceous glands originate in the epidermis and extend downward into the dermis below. Epidermal specifics are developed and maintained through interaction between the epidermis and dermis and distribution of papillae in the superficial layer of the dermis (Fig. 3).

The dermis

The dermis, also known as the corium or true skin, consists of a matrix of stratified connective tissue composed of fibrous proteins – collagen, elastin and reticulin fibers – and an 'amorphous ground substance'.[6] The connective tissue layers are aligned at various angles to one another, providing it with the capability of adapting to the continuous movements of the body. The two major strata of the dermis are (1) a reticular layer composed of a network of thick collagen fibers intermingled with the elastic fibers (elastin) and other components; and (2) the papillary layer, where the collagen fibers form a loose, three dimensional, irregular network. The collagen provides the resistance to mechanical stress and elastin can be compared to rubber because of its ability to stretch and easily resume its shape.

The characteristics of the papillary layer are the highly sensitive and vascular papillae, which are minute conical projections which have round or blunted extremities. They are formed by the elastin fibers that rise perpendicularly from the surface of the reticular layer to the epidermis, extend to penicillate formations until they form a globular end, which pushes against the basal layer and indents the inner surface of the epidermis. These fibers anchor the epidermis to the dermis and determine the pattern of the skin. On the general surface of the body, which is smooth, they are few in number and are exceedingly small. In the palms of the hands and soles of the feet, they are large, closely aggregated together, and are arranged in parallel curved lines, forming the elevated ridges seen on the outer surface of the skin, i.e., the fingerprints and footprints. Each ridge contains two rows of papillae, and between the rows the ducts of the sweat glands pass outwards to open on the tops of the ridges.

The dermis, which is tough, flexible and highly elastic, varies in thickness from less than 0.5 mm on the eyelid to 3 mm or more on the palms and soles, and constitutes from 15% to 20% of total body weight.[6,7,9] By binding considerable amounts of water, it represents a water storage organ.[7]

Except for the arrector pili muscles attached to the hair follicles, the dermis is relatively free of muscles. However, the skin from the areola and nipple of the breast, penis, scrotum and perineum contains variable numbers of smooth muscle fibers which, when contracted, produce wrinkling.

The panniculus adiposus or subcutaneous tissue

Below the dermis resides a thick layer of connective tissue, specialized in the formation and storage of fat. The variably thick fatty layer of tissue serves as heat insulation, a depot of energy, as well as a mechanical shock-absorber for the underlying tissue. This layer is considerably thicker in women and is the reason for the finer and softer texture of their skin.[5] It is also a major factor in wrinkling – the loss of the supporting layer of fat that accompanies aging or sudden weight loss causes the outer layer of skin, which does not shrink at the same rate, to sag and fold into wrinkles.[2]

The panniculus adiposus contains larger blood vessels, lymphatics, and nerves. The lymphatics, less known, but probably as extensive in number as the blood vessels, serve as a drainage system to remove water, proteins and other materials from the extracellular environment of the dermis.

THE SWEAT GLANDS

The body continuously produces heat by oxidation of fats and carbohydrates and the skin functions much the same as a radiator-surface, giving up heat which is brought to the surface via the blood through the rich, complex vascular network found in the dermis. The vascularity of the human skin is so rich that it is able to store 4.5% of the body's total blood volume. The center for control of this regulating system (basal metabolism) is located in the hypothalamic center of the brain. In order to maintain a constant body temperature (98.6° F; 37° C), body heat must be continuously adjusted. To aid the skin as a cooling device, sweat glands pour water on its surface, and evaporation absorbs heat from the skin. Without the sweat glands to dissipate heat and thus cool the body, it would burn up.

There are two types of sweat glands: (1) the eccrine glands, which are not associated with the hair follicle, and (2) the apocrine glands, which are.

The eccrine glands

Eccrine sweat glands are simple tubes, consisting of a secretory coil (body) lodged in the dermis, and a straight duct that opens onto the epidermis and discharges sweat. These glands are of major importance to the body's thermal regulation because evaporation of the sweat they excrete helps to reduce body temperature. Humans have from two to four million of these glands distributed over almost every part of the body, but they are more numerous in the palms of the hands, soles of the feet, and the forehead. Only the glans penis, clitoris, labia minora and the inner surface of the prepuce have no eccrine glands.

The sweating process is continuous, even though at times the skin appears to be dry because the sweat evaporates as soon as it is formed. The total output of these glands can be enormous: as much as 10 liters per day.[10] They not only respond to heat-stimuli, sweating is also induced by emotional stress due to nervousness or excitement, but in these instances is confined to the palms, axillae, soles and forehead. They also serve as excretory organs to discharge wastes, such as organic compounds and 'heavy metals'.[11]

The apocrine glands

The apocrine glands are mainly located in the axillary and genital areas, and secrete only small amounts of lipids over long intervals. Because these glands do not become functional before puberty, it is assumed that they are hormone-influenced.

The secretory part of the apocrine glands rests in the dermis, but those of the larger ones extend into the subcutaneous tissue. They have a straight narrow duct that runs parallel to the hair follicle and usually opens into the pilosebaceous canal above the entrance of the sebaceous glands, but some ducts open directly upon the surface of the skin. These glands are not as physiologically important as the eccrine glands, and their secretion produces the perspiration odor so repugnant to man. It is a natural human attribute and Montagna believes that in the past this odorous secretion may have played a role in the chemical communication of earliest man:[6] some odors attract, others repell. In our modern society, many products on store shelves owe their very existence to these glands.

THE PILOSEBACEOUS UNIT

The hair follicle and one or more sebaceous (oil) glands attached to it comprise the pilosebaceous unit. Each hair consists of a root, the part implanted in the skin, and a shaft, the portion projecting above the surface of the skin. The sebaceous glands secrete an oily substance called sebum, which lubricates the hairs and the skin. This is the most accepted function of sebum; some authors believe it prevents fungal or bacterial infection and helps to maintain the acid mantle of the skin; others believe it is useless and even harmful. Scientists still do not have the final answer.

The sebaceous glands

The sebaceous glands are sacculated lobules, sebum-secreting structures, lodged in the dermis. Most of these glands develop from the follicle epithelium in the fetal stage, and are located at its upper part. They are found in most parts of the skin, except in the palms of the hands or soles of the feet. They are especially abundant in the scalp, forehead, face, and anogenital area. Each sebaceous gland consists of a unilobular or multi-branched cluster of acini (lobules), connected to a common excretory duct. Each acinus is composed of a rounded mass of cells, in which the outer layer of undifferentiated, compressed basal cells rests against the basement membrane. These cells differentiate lipid (sebum vacuoles) in a centripetal direction. Sebaceous differentiation is the synthesis, secretion and accumulation of lipid (sebum vacuoles), resulting in a progressive enlargement and deformation of the cells toward the center where they finally rupture. The lipid of these cells, together with their debris (cellular remnants) form the sebum which is spilled into the duct of the glands. The ducts open most frequently into the hair follicles, but occasionally upon the surface of the skin.

Sebaceous glands are structurally, grossly, and microscopically similar, but vary in size, activity, and response to trophic agents (nutrition, etc.), according to their location in the body, as well as among individuals, ethnic groups, and according to sex and age.[6] Some authors conclude that they are smaller in women than in men; others believe they are large in both sexes, although sebum production is commonly less in women than in men.[12]

In general, the size of the sebaceous glands varies inversely with that of the hair follicles to which they are attached. Both sebaceous glands and hair follicles are large in the skin of the scalp, eyebrows and eyelashes. The largest ones are located in the skin of the face, forehead, neck, upper back, shoulders and upper arm, the scrotum and anogenital regions, and are associated with vellus hair. Some contain brush-like tufts of vellus hair that remain in the follicle when a new hair is formed. To classify these enormous glands, they are given the name 'sebaceous follicles' because of their 'anatomical peculiarities': they have a relatively small hair rudiment, large, lobulated sebaceous gland acini and a wide infundibulum (funnel-shaped passage) filled with 'horn cell' material.

At puberty, sebaceous glands also develop in the smooth, bare border or junction of the pinkish-red area of the lips and the surrounding skin, and are more numerous in the upper than in the lower lip. They can also differentiate in other organs; for example, numerous glands are present between the lactiferous ducts at the tip of the breast nipple in both men and women.

It is also at puberty when the common teenage complexion problems of blackheads (comedones), pimples and acne begins. The onset of these conditions coincides with the physiologic increase in sex hormone production in both males and females as they enter puberty. The size and rate of growth of the sebaceous glands are regulated by hormones; they are very sensitive to androgens which expedite the maturing of these glands during puberty.

Blackheads are the earliest lesions of common acne and are associated with hypersecretion of sebum and thickening of the hair follicle. Acne vulgaris, which occurs only in the presence of a blackhead, is a multi-factorial disease which develops in the sebaceous follicle. The disease is not solely due to the amount of sebum produced by the sebaceous glands, but to an alteration in the process of keratinization as well. The follicle plug consists of loose cells, sebum and bacteria, and the free fatty acid fraction of sebum is considered to be important in the cause of inflammation. The pigment of the follicle orifice has been identified as melanin.

The hair follicle

Each hair, consisting of a root (the part implanted in the skin) and a shaft (the portion projecting above the surface of the skin) grows out of a follicle. Hair follicles are tube-like appendages of the epidermis that slant downward into the dermis; the longest ones extend into the underlying subcutaneous tissue (panniculus adiposus), where they form their greatest diameter, the bulb (Fig. 4). The hair bulb is moulded over a cone of connective tissue, the papilla, which is continuous with the dermic layer of the follicle. Large papillae are supplied with a large number of blood vessels; smaller ones have less, or they are not visible. The blood vessels provide nourishment for the growing hair (Fig. 5). From the center outwards, the growing hair is surrounded by the follicle, which consists of the inner and outer root sheath, and the connective tissue sheath.

1.   *The inner root sheath* consists of (1) a cuticle next to the hair, which is composed of a single layer of flattened, imbricated scales with their free edges directed downward, which interlock with the cuticle cells of the hair shaft which grow upward; (2) one or two layers (two in the larger follicles of men) of flattened cells, known as Huxley's layer; (3) a single layer of cubical cells, which become elongated vertically in the upper bulb, called Henle's layer. Above the center of the follicle all three layers become fused into a solid hyalin layer. The cells of the Henle's layer are keratinized immediately after they rise from the matrix, and slide easily upward against the cells of the outer root sheath. The main function of the inner root sheath is thought to be to shape the hair.[6]

2.   *The outer root sheath* covers the inner root sheath. Its upper half is the

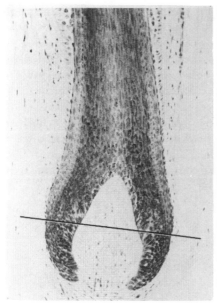 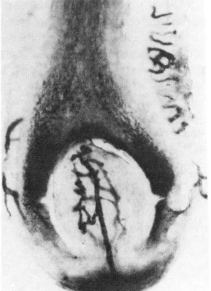

Figure 4. Longitudinal section through the bulb of a scalp terminal hair follicle. The black line separates the upper from the lower bulb at the critical level. (From: IBID)

Figure 5. A tuft of blood vessels inside the dermal papilla of an eyebrow follicle demonstrated with the alkaline phosphatase technique. (From: IBID)

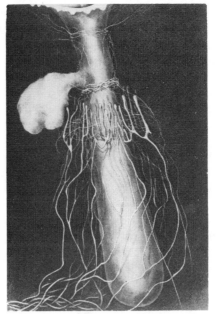

Figure 6. Diagram of the disposition of nerves around a small hair follicle. (From: IBID)

stable portion of the follicle and the continuation of the epidermis. The lower half is the transition portion, and during catagen forms the hair germ and epithelial sac, which supplies the seeds for the next generation of hairs.[6] The outer root sheath and the epidermal cells are basically similar, but have some difference in their components. The mitotic activity common in the follicle, where the outer root sheath and the epidermis blend, often presents an electrologist with difficulties.[15]. The cells forming the keratinized surface layer are constantly sloughed off and can build up, often blocking the follicle opening.

The outer root sheath can be divided into three segments: (a) the lower part around the bulb which is only one or two cells thick; (b) the middle part from the neck of the bulb to the level of the sebaceous glands, which has three layers of cells that store large amounts of glycogen (animal starch). These cells are reduced to flimsy, spongy sacs in the middle third of the follicle and contain more glycogen than the others.[6] The electrologist's current makes greater use of the moisture at this level. (c) The third portion of the outer root sheath extends above the entrance of the sebaceous glands and is called the pilary canal. The uneven thickness of the outer root sheath of large follicles causes the hair to grow eccentrically. Its overall thickness is proportional to the size of the hair follicle – large hairs have large outer root sheaths.[6]

3.   The connective tissue components surrounding the follicle are made up of three layers. The innermost layer, the hyaline membrane (vitreous membrane, basement membrane), which is thick around the lower third of the follicle, but thin in the upper portion. The middle layer consists of compact fibers arranged circularly around the follicle. The outermost layer consists of a thick stratum of connective tissue, arranged in longitudinal bundles; it is attached by a stalk to the dermal papilla at the base of the follicle and is continuous with the papillary layer of the dermis.

Connected to the hair follicles are minute bundles of smooth muscular fibers, termed arrector pili muscles. They arise from the surface layer of the dermis and are attached to the hair follicle below the entrance of the sebaceous gland duct. Activated by nerves, they contract when one is subjected to chills or fright and pull the hair shaft to a 'stand-up' position; the skin around the follicle is drawn into elevations known as 'goose pimples' (Fig. 6).

The hair shaft

The hair that projects above the surface of the skin is a dead structure; it is composed of keratinized cells which are compactly cemented together. The term keratin originates from the Greek word keras, meaning 'horny'. The hair shaft consists, from the center outwards, of a medulla, cortex and cuticle (Fig. 7).

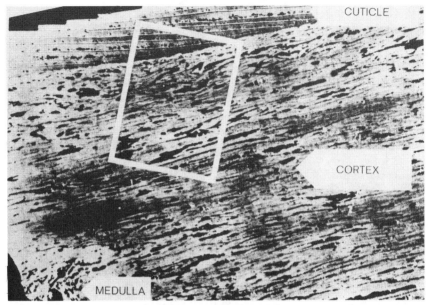

Figure 7. Micrograph of the inner structure of hair, using Electron microscopy (EM), magnified 3,000 times. A small portion of the medulla can be seen at the lower left; the cortex covers the center portion and the cuticle is at the top. (Courtesy of the Wella International Research Department, from their publication *On the Structure of Human Hair,* Darmstadt, West Germany, p 6)

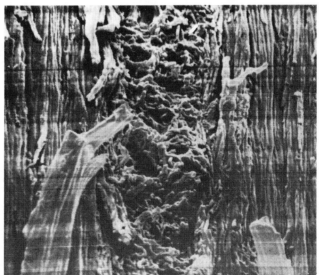

Figure 8. An SEM micrograph (magnified 2,000 times) showing the medulla which is buried within the numerous cables of the cortex. Note that the structure of the medulla is not uniform: some sections appear to be made of short, tangled pieces of fiber; others seem almost saucer or plate-like in appearance. Voids are also evident. (From: IBID, p 28)

The medulla is the central axis of the hair and is composed of large, loosely connected keratinized cells; it may be continuous, disjointed, or absent. In fine hair it is usually absent. Figure 8 is a micrograph of the medulla, cortex and cuticle, magnified 2,000 times, which reveals that the structure of the medulla is not uniform; some sections appear to be made of short, tangled pieces of fiber; other sections seem almost plate or saucer-like in appearance. The voids or air spaces between the cells are also evident. These air spaces greatly determine the sheen and color tones of the hair by influencing the reflection of light.

The cortex constitutes the bulk of the hair, and in pigmented hair contains melanin granules which are imbedded between the keratinized thread-like structural fibers. Figure 9a-c shows three micrographic views of the cortex. Figure 9a depicts a flap of hair lifted to reveal the long-threadlike structural elements of the cortex. Figure 9b reveals a closer view of the fibers and shows that they do not lie parallel to each other, but are twisted and cross each other. They are not randomly placed, but through weaving and interlacing, the lengthwise oriented fibers are spun into a cable much like cotton into a thread. In spite of the conformity of the individual fibers, a degree of entanglement results which leads to the overall strength and elasticity of the hair. Figure 9c reveals the amorphous substance which covers the fibers. Between the fibers are delicate air spaces called 'fusis', and in the living portion of the follicle, these fusis are filled with fluid. As the hair grows upward, they dry out and air replaces the fluid.

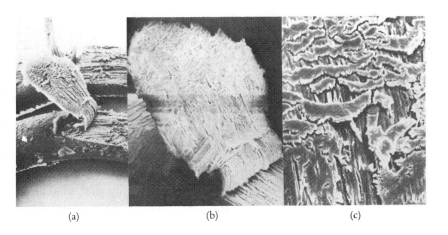

(a)   (b)   (c)

Figure 9.   Three views of the cortex. (a) an SEM micrograph (magnified 200 times) shows a hair with a split section and flap lifted up to reveal the cortex. (b) An SEM micrograph, (magnified 400 times) of the same section. (c) An SEM micrograph (magnified 2,000 times) which clearly shows an amorphous mass covering the thread-like longitudinal cortex fibers. (From: IBID, p 16)

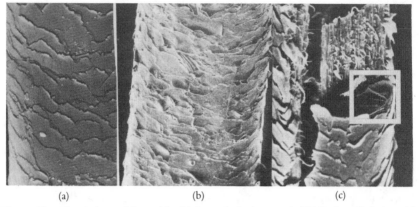

(a)   (b)   (c)

Figure 10. Three views of the cuticle. (a) An optical microscopic (OM) view of a hair cuticle magnified 1,000 times. (b) An SEM micrograph, magnified 1,000 times. (c) An SEM micrograph (magnified 1,000 times) which clearly shows that the cuticle of the hair consists of several thicknesses of thin, curved layers. In this micrograph, nine layers were noted. In all three views, note that the edges of the cuticle are loose and do not lie completely flat. (From: IBID)

The cuticle consists of several thicknesses of thin, curved, overlapping layers that appear cylindrical in shape. These layers are held together by a 'cement-like' substance. In healthy hair, it is very elastic and firmly bonded together. Brushing, combing, handling, or abuse causes the cuticle to be worn away, and as the edges of the cuticle loosen, small elongated fragments often detach. The shape of the fragments helped to further the popular belief in the past that the cuticle was composed of 'fish-like' scales or shingles (Fig. 10a–c). In the past it was believed that the cuticle consisted of only one to three layers, but SEM micrographs have revealed as many as 12 layers. The cuticle cells are free of pigments and are translucent. By interlocking with the inner root sheath cuticle, the cuticle cells of the hair shaft anchor the hair in the follicle.

THE PHYSIOLOGY OF HAIR GROWTH

Between the second and third month of fetal life, follicles appear on the eyebrows, chin and upper lip; slightly later they appear on the scalp and forehead. During the fourth and fifth gestational month they spread throughout the body in a cephalocaudal progression. Follicle development over the body is complete by the eighth fetal month and the primary (lanugo) hairs are shed.

The hair follicles are formed during embryonic development by an interaction between the epidermal and dermal components of the skin. The crowding of basal cells in the still undifferentiated epidermis and the concentration of mesodermal cells (future papilla) are the first stage of development.

These hair germ cells grow downward as a solid column into the dermis, passing through various stages in which sebaceous glands and the arrector pili muscles begin to develop. After all components of the pilosebaceous units have been established, the bulb encloses the dermal papilla. The inner root sheath differentiates first and forms a cone, below which the cortical cells of the hair are formed. At this time, the pilary canal through which the first hair emerges has been established.

After a period of growth, the hair goes into a period of rest (telogen). The postnatal behavior of the follicle is established as early as four and a half to five months gestation, except for the scalp follicles. They appear to grow without cyclic activity and are all at anagen phase (growing) at birth. Within the first few days of life, the hair follicles enter a telogen phase and the mosaic pattern of the follicle activity is established six to twelve weeks later, in which each hair enters the anagen and subsequent phases of telogen and anagen independent of each other. No new follicles develop in adult skin and follicle distribution is the same in both sexes.

The growth cycle

The hair growth cycle involves two main phases, anagen (active growth) and telogen (resting phase), as well as a transition period (catagen). Throughout the three growth phases, the follicle has a changing anatomy which involves the lower or transition portion.[6] The follicle's upper portion is stable and permanent. During anagen, the transition portion of the follicle is built up; during catagen, it is broken down; in telogen, the anatomy of the dormant follicle is incomplete. Figure 11 depicts a diagram of the growing hair follicle and indicates the various regions to be discussed in the text. Figures 12, 13, and 14 illustrate the hair growth cycle.

The anagen phase or active growth period can be divided into two segments: (1) the reconstruction of the hair bulb, and (2) growth of the hair. The early phase is signaled by mitotic activity of the hair germ. Mitotic activity is the continuous process of cell division: one cell divides into two cells, two into four, and so on. Through this activity, the hair germ grows and builds a solid cord that extends deeper into the dermis to surround the papilla and form a new onion-shaped bulb. The bulb is the thickest part of the follicle and consists of the lower third of the follicle, which is short when the bulb is formed. At the widest diameter of the dermal papilla, the 'critical level', investigators have separated the bulb into two regions: the lower part consisting of the matrix; the upper part of the bulb, the place of cell differentiation.

The matrix, or intercellular material of a tissue, is the basic substance from which all living organisms are made. In the case of the hair follicle, the matrix is the busy cell mass on the circumference of the dermal papilla. The volume of the follicle matrix is approximately ten times that of the dermal papilla.[16]

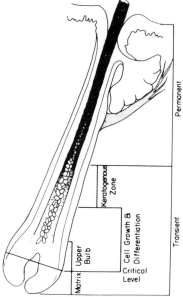

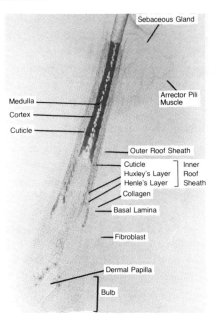

Figure 11. Diagram of a growing hair follicle indicating the various regions discussed in the text. (From: Montagna, W. and Parakkal, P. F., *The Structure and Function of Skin.* New York, Academic Press, 1974).

Figure 12. Diagram showing a growing (anagen) terminal hair follicle. Note the complex, relative position of the various layers. (From: IBID)

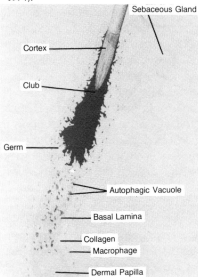

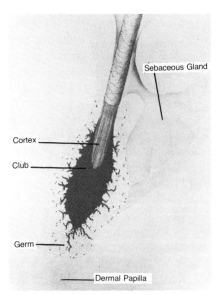

Figure 13. Diagram of a follicle in the transitional state (catagen). Note the corrugation of the basal lamina and the resorption of the epithelial and connective tissue elements. (From: IBID)

Figure 14. Diagram of a quiescent (telogen) terminal hair follicle. Note the relationship between the club and the germ. The dermal papilla is now outside the follicle. (From: IBID)

The mitotic activity of the matrix cells is very strong, each cell dividing about every 13 hours. The matrix cells on top of the papilla build the medulla of the hair; those from the sides of the papilla form the cortex; and those from the neck of the papilla shape the hair cuticle and inner root sheath. Some mitotic activity is also found in the upper or permanent part of the bulb where cells grow and differentiate.

As the new cells move up into the upper part of the bulb, they form the hair shaft and inner root sheath, growing many times their original size before emerging into the pre-keratinization zone, and move further up into the keratogenous zone. In the upper part of the bulb, melanocytes supply the cells of the cortex and medulla with melanin granules to give the hair its color. The upward directing cells of the hair shaft cuticle, and the downward pointing cuticle cells of the inner root sheath are interlocked and travel together. In the widened portion of the pilosebaceous canal, the inner root sheath of the follicle forms a loose hyalin collar around the emerging hair. The inner root sheath is dissolved in the pilary canal, probably through chemical reaction; however, no detailed information is available. Before the hair shaft emerges on the surface of the skin, it is lubricated with sebum produced by the sebaceous glands.

During the *anagen* phase, production of the hair is continuous until the growing hair has reached its full length. The duration of this phase differs according to location on the body, and ranges from a few weeks in the fingers, four to six months in the thigh, to three to eight years in the scalp.[6,17]

The catagen phase. When the growing hair has reached its full length, the anagen phase ends and catagen begins with the cessation of melanin production of the melanocytes in the upper part of the bulb. The tip of the dermal papilla shortens and the matrix ceases to form the medulla. Consequently, the lower part of the still growing hair becomes lighter, or white, and unmedullated. Next, the papilla shrinks, and the formation of the inner root sheath ceases before the mitotic activity comes to a complete halt. No new cells are formed, but the cortex cells continue to move upwards from the bulb, differentiate and keratinize to form the non-pigmented catagen hair.

The bulb, depleted of its cells, consists only of the outer root sheath which collapses from a hollow tube to a solid epithelial column of cells to which the released papilla is attached.[18] Gradual absorption of these cells from below forms the hair germ and results in the ascent of the papilla. The vitreous membrane thickens and corrugates; the connective tissue becomes wrinkled, collapses and fills the path vacated by the bulb. The last step of the catagen follicle is the building of the club. The lower end of the catagen hair becomes keratinized and builds the hair club which is anchored into the germ-sac. The epithelial or germ sac is described as two or three layers of germ cells which surround the club. The cells of the germ sac are the seeds for the next generation of hair, and are the most important part of the dormant follicle or telogen phase.[6]

The telogen phase. The hair follicle in the telogen phase has only about one-half to one-third of the length of a growing follicle. The deepest extension is entirely within the dermis. The characteristic structures of a follicle in telogen are the club and the hair germ. The cells of the shrunken papilla are arranged in a ball, resting at the base of the hair germ. After a time of rest, a new hair root is regenerated from the hair germ (also called a secondary germ) and with increased mitotic activity grows downward, and the whole cycle begins again with the anagen phase. Some of the club hairs formed during catagen may fall out in telogen but, mostly, they are shed in the early part of the anagen phase as the new hair shaft approaches the surface of the skin.

Most biologists are convinced that the dermal papilla induces the regeneration of the hair follicles, and Hinkel states that this has also been the traditional opinion of electrologists.[15] However, experiments on rat vibrissae have shown that if the dermal papilla is surgically removed, a new one may be formed. The phenomenon of axillary hair regrowth after subcutaneous tissue shaving (surgical tissue removal of layers under the dermis) encouraged investigations by Inaba and his co-workers.[19] They studied tissue in which the hair bulb (papilla and matrix) and most of the follicle up to the level of the sebaceous duct had been removed. Both the dermal papilla of the anagen hair and the telogen hair was eliminated. Six months after surgery new young hairs were formed. The regeneration of the hair follicles occurred from the outer root sheath remnants, but only when the sebaceous glands were preserved. The new papilla was reconstructed from a mass of mesenchymal cells. They further stated that postoperative hair follicle formation is different from the ordinary hair cycle and must be considered as new hair growth, because it has stages similar to, but not identical with, fetal hair formation.

To initiate a new anagen phase in the telogen follicle, Chase et al described plucking as the stimulating physical agent. The method was applied in animal experiments to produce an even growth of hair, and although cutting and shaving have no effect on the hair cycle, and do not stimulate new growth, they observed that dekeratinizing depilatory agents, such as barium sulfide, do have an influence. Except for the loss of the hair shaft, there is no effect on the growing (anagen) follicle; on the telogen follicle, it has the same effect as plucking.

Classification of hair types

There are three types of human hair:

1. Lanugo hair, which is the fur-like primary hair covering the fetus which is shed before birth, and in rare instances afterward. This hair is

extremely fine, soft, unmedullated and usually not pigmented.

2.   Vellus hair, replaces the fur-like, ultrafine lanugo hair which covered the body during fetal development. It is soft, unmedullated, rarely pigmented, and normally grows less than 2 cm long.

3.   Terminal hair, which is longer, coarser, pigmented, and medullated, replaces vellus hairs at specific sites of the body and at specific times of life. Terminal hairs have a wide range of caliber and length in a given area, as well as a wider range from one area of the body to another. Vellus hairs are often situated in a satellite position to terminal hairs.[25]

Hairs vary in length, thickness and color on different parts of the body, as well as in different sexes and races. In some parts of the skin, such as the eyelids, the hairs are so short they do not project far beyond the follicles that contain them; other hairs, such as scalp hair, grow considerably long; the eyelashes, eyebrows, beard and pubic hair grow remarkably thick.

Although hair cannot be strictly classified on the basis of length or thickness, because there are so many variables, there are some basic characteristics according to location of growth on the body:

1.   Scalp hair, which exhibits many form variations, may grow to 36 inches, but longer lengths have been reported. The diameter of scalp hair increases rapidly during the first three or four years after birth, less during the next six years, and scarcely after age 12.

2.   Eyelashes and eyebrows are curved and flattened, and grow about 1 cm long. Except in very blond and fair skinned persons, the eyelashes are the darkest hairs on the body.

3.   Body hair, both vellus and terminal, has a fine, long tip. Growth of terminal body hair can reach up to 6 cm in length.

4.   Beard and mustache hairs, the coarsest on the body, have a blunt tip, and a larger root than head hair. They grow 0.27 mm per day if uncut and can grow as long as 30 cm.

5.   Pubic hair, which is coarse, irregular, and asymmetrical, can be curved, straight, or spiral tufted and reach a length of up to 6 cm. Pubic hairs are almost always curled around their axis and in a woman grow in an inverted triangular pattern; in men the pattern is rhomboidal.

6.   Axillary (underarm) hair is curled or twisted around its axis. Its length varies between 1 and 60 mm.[6]

The difference in size and length of each hair is determined by the size of the follicle, which in turn is determined by the papilla from which it grows and the depth to which the follicle extends into the dermic tissue. The deeper the follicle extends into the dermis, the longer the hair growth. Short thick hairs have a larger follicle and a more shallow penetration into the skin.

It is estimated that approximately 18% of terminal hairs grow singly, the rest in clusters of three, but groups of two or four (rarely five) are also found. The average depth to which the terminal hair follicle extends into the dermis is about 3.5 mm. Vellus hair follicles situated in satellite positions around the terminal hair follicle extend to only about 0.5 mm below the skin's surface. Hair grows an average of 0.3 to 0.4 mm per day, or three-quarters of an inch per month, and grows faster between ages 15 and 30. In young women, hair growth is greatest between ages 16 and 24, when a growth of seven inches per year has been noted. The growth rate slows down and density decreases between ages 50 and 60. Approximately 90% of the 100,000-150,000 scalp hairs are said to be growing, an average of 10% are resting, and about 100 club hairs are shed each day.

References

1. Cooper, W., *Hair: Sex, Society, Symbolism*. New York, Stein and Day, 1971
2. Bluefarb, S. M., The skin and its disorders. In, Family Medical Guide New York, Meredith Press, 1966
3. Stuttgen, G., Welcome Address, Lectures and discussions of a symposium. In, *Androgeniza-tion in Women: Acne, Seborrhoea, Androgenetic Alopecia and Hirsutism*. Hammerstein, J., Lachnit-Fixon, U. and Neumann, F. et al (eds). Amsterdam, Excerpta Medica, 1980, p 3
4. Fitzpatrick, T. B., *Dermatology in General Medicine*. Fitzpatrick, T. B., Eisen, A. Z., Wolff, K., et al (eds). New York, McGraw-Hill, 1979
5. Zacarian, S. A., *Your Skin, its Problems and Care*. Radnor, P. A., Chilton Book Co, 1973
6. Montagna, W. and Parakkal, P. F., *The Structure and Function of Skin*. New York, Academic Press, 1974
7. Breathnach, A. S. and Wolff, K., In, *Dermatology in General Medicine*, Fitzpatrick, et al (eds). New York, McGraw-Hill, 1979
8. Cohen, A., *Handbook of Microscopic Anatomy for the Health Sciences*. St. Louis, C. V. Mosby, 1975
9. Bevelander, G. and Ramaley, J. A., *Essentials of Histology*. St. Louis, C. V. Mosby, 1979
10. Sato, K., In, *Dermatology in General Medicine*. Fitzpatrick, et al (eds). New York, McGraw-Hill, 1979
11. Robertshaw, D., In, *Dermatology in General Medicine*. (IBID)
12. Strauss, J. S., In, *Hair Research, Status and Future Aspects*. Orfanos, C. C., Montagna, W. and Stuttgen, G., (eds). Berlin, Springer Verlag, 1981
13. Luderschmidt, C., Pathogenesis of acne vulgaris. In, *Androgenization in Women: Acne, Seborrhoea, Androgenetic Alopecia and Hirsutism*. Amsterdam, Excerpta Medica, 1980, p 77
14. Strauss, J. S., In, *Dermatology in General Medicine*. Fitzpatrick, T. B., et al (eds). St. Louis, McGraw-Hill, 1979
15. Hinkel, A. R. and Lind, R. W., *Electrolysis, Thermolysis and the Blend*. Arroway Publ., California, 1968
16. Montagna, W., *The Structure and Function of Skin*. New York, Academic Press, 1962
17. Ebling, F. J., In, *Hair Research, Status and Future Aspects*. Orfanos, C. E., Montagna, W. and Stuttgen, G., (eds). Berlin, Springer Verlag, 1981
18. Pinkus, H., In, *Hair Trace Elements and Human Illness*, Brown, A. C. and Crounse, R. G., (eds). New York, Praeger Publishers, 1980
19. Inaba, H., Anthony, J. and McKinstry, C., Histologic study of the regeneration of axillary hair after removal with subcutaneous tissue shaver. J. Invest Dermatol 72:244, 1979
20. Chase, H. B., In, *The Biology of Hair Growth*. Montagna, W., Ellis, R. A. (eds). New York, Academic Press, 1958

21. Ravin, J. G. and Hodge, G. P., Hypertrichosis portrayed in art. JAMA 207:533, 1969
22. Turner, as quoted by Hegedus, S. I. and Schorr, W. F., Acquired hypertrichosis lanuginosa and malignancy. Arch Derm 106:84, 1972
23. Van Scott, E. J., Physiology of hair growth. Clin Obstet Gynecol 7:1062, 1964
24. Savill, A. and Warren C., *The Hair and Scalp*. Baltimore, Williams and Wilkins, 1962
25. Bates, G. W., Hirsutism and androgen excess in childhood and adolescence. Ped Clin N Am 28:513, (May) 1981

4
Hirsutism and the Endocrine System

P. K. Natrajan, M.D.

The terms hirsutism and hypertrichosis are both used to describe excessive hair growth in the female, which, cosmetically, is one of the most disturbing complaints in women. Though the terms are used synonymously, and it is often hard to tell the difference between the two conditions, there is a definite difference. In hirsutism, there is an increase in the cyclic growth, rate of growth, and diameter of hormone dependent terminal hairs on areas of the body, especially the face, where terminal hairs are usually quite small in caliber and length, and are not easily distinguishable from vellus hairs. In hypertrichosis, there is an overgrowth of both vellus and terminal hairs over the entire body surface; the hairs grow longer and faster than normal, but are not increased in diameter and are not limited to a masculine pattern of growth, as in hirsutism.

By definition, hirsutism refers only to the female because of the facial and masculine hair growth pattern, which is the normal pattern of the male. Facial hair growth may range from a few fuzzy hairs to a full beard that the patient must shave every day. Hirsutism is caused by either an increased sensitivity of the hair follicle to normal levels of androgen hormones in the blood stream (termed primary or idiopathic hirsutism), or is due to increased androgen production by the endocrine glands, i.e., the adrenals and ovaries (termed secondary or true hirsutism). Primary hirsutism has an onset at puberty with hair growth increasing until the third decade of life, when it stabilizes (Fig. 1). True hirsutism begins either before or after puberty due to an endocrine disorder which causes increased secretion by the glands (Fig. 2).

Hypertrichosis, on the other hand, can occur in either males or females.

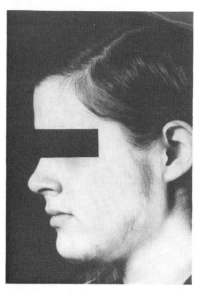

Figure 1. Adolescent female with increased facial hair growth.

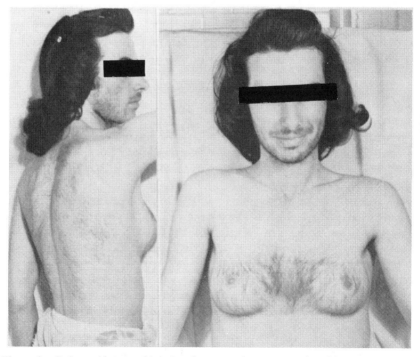

Figure 2. Patient with severe hirsutism due to ovarian tumor (arrhenoblastoma). (Courtesy of Novak, E. R., Virilizing tumors of the ovary, in, *The Hirsute Female*, R. B. Greenblatt (ed). Springfield, IL., Charles C. Thomas, 1963, pp 195-210)

This type of hair growth is considered to be a genetic or racial trait, or a constitutional variation in follicle sensitivity, and not due to a systemic disorder.

In order to understand the development of these two conditions, it is important to point out that genetic predisposition and endocrine factors control a wide range of possibilities in each human's development. Though no difference exists in the hair follicle distribution between the male and female, their sex-specific hair patterns are determined by genetic predisposition, which in turn affects the nature and amounts of hormones produced by the endocrine glands that influence the type and extent of hair follicle response in various areas of the body.[1] Endocrine hormones influence, modify, and stimulate growth at the hair follicle cells to produce the pattern, quantity, texture, and distribution of body hair.

Hair can be classified into three hormonal types: (1) genetic hair present at birth, influenced by changes in growth hormone production but not dependent on steroid (sex) hormones, is known as *asexual hair*. This type includes head hair, eyebrows, eyelashes, hair on the distal portions of the arms and legs, midphalangel areas, and to some extent lumbosacral hair. (2) Hair growth that develops in both male and female alike at puberty under the influence of increased adrenal and gonadal androgen production is known as *ambisexual hair*. This hormonal type includes pubic, axillary, lower limbs, and lower abdomen hairs. (3) Hair that is influenced by increased amounts of androgen hormone production by the gonads is known as *true sexual hair*. This type includes the beard, mustache, nasal passage, external ear, and body hairs, especially on the back, and is more pronounced in the male due to larger amounts of testosterone production by the testicles. In the male, testosterone levels are 15-30% higher than in the female, and terminal hairs in these areas on the female body are hard to distinguish from vellus hairs.

Of the endocrine glands, the adrenals, testes, ovaries and placenta are specialized for the conversion of cholesterol into biologically active steroid hormones, i.e., corticosteroids, estrogens, progestogens, and androgens.[2] Cholesterol, the parent compound, is metabolized to pregnenolone, which is the common substrate and serves as the immediate precursor for the synthesis of all hormonal steroids through various metabolic pathways (Fig. 3). The action of steroids is mediated through cytosol receptors – sex hormone binding globulin (SHBG) and albumin – to which they are bound and carried through the blood stream for conversion in the various target tissues, which include the skin, pilosebaceous unit, and central nervous system. Receptor steroid complexes bind to target cell nuclei where they activate genes for steroid specific proteins and are then transferred to the nucleus of the cell. All tissues that respond to androgen administration contain measurable cytosol androgen-receptor protein.[3]

Initiation of new hair growth is due to stimulation and transformation of existing follicles by the entrance of androgens to cells where they undergo a

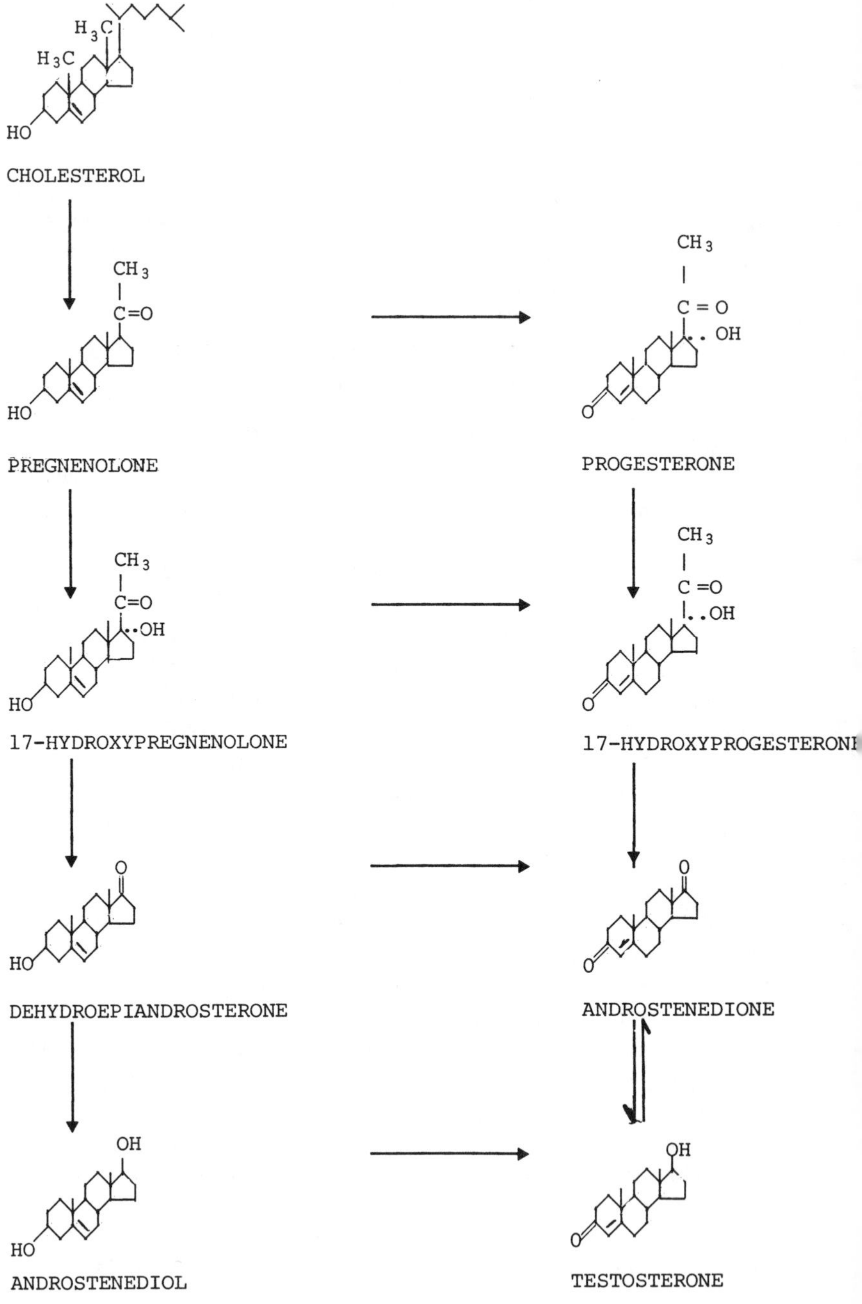

Figure 3.   Pathways in the formation of androgens with structural formulas.

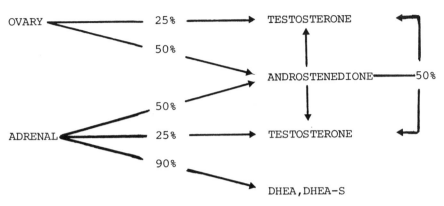

Figure 4. Sources of androgens and the relative contribution of the ovary and adrenal glands.

series of conversions that lead to testosterone and dihydrotestosterone (DHT); testosterone and DHT are bound to specific cytoplasmic receptor proteins, which then are transferred to the nuclei, where testosterone (the proandrogen) is converted to DHT (the actual androgen).[2] The other androgens must first be converted to testosterone or DHT because they do not bind firmly to the receptor. The receptor-steroid complex enters the nucleus where it binds to DNA, and leads to the formation of messenger RNA, which then initiates the formation of a new protein through ribosomal RNA, thus stimulating hair growth. Hirsutism occurs when the intracellular metabolism of the hair follicle is changed, either at the receptor site or the nuclear site by hypersecretion of androgens by the adrenals and ovaries.

Other hormones, such as corticoids, thyroid, growth hormone, and estrogens, influence and modify hair without stimulating growth. The diameter of hair and rate of growth are also hormonally affected: androgens and growth hormone increase, and estrogens decrease size and growth rate. Furthermore, though estrogens do not stimulate growth, they can prolong the growth cycle once it has been initiated.

Although androgens are produced in larger quantities by the male testes and are primarily thought of as 'male' hormones, they are essential for the development and maintenance of a balanced hormonal milieu in the reproductive female as well. They regulate, modify, and stimulate many mechanisms in both sexes: protein anabolism, the growth and function of the male genitals, secondary sex characteristics of the male, sperm production, stimulation of sexual hair growth, and they are the immediate precursor for the formation of female sex hormones. The principal androgens produced by the adrenal are dehydroepiandrosterone (DHEA) and dehydroepiandrosterone sulfate (DHEA-S). The ovary converts nonandrogenic C_{21} steroids (pregnenolone and progesterone) into androgenic steroids (androstenedione and testosterone) which then convert to estrogens. Estrogens limit the physiologic action of testosterone by increasing its protein-binding capacity and thereby limiting the amount of free testosterone in the blood stream to be converted to dihydrotestosterone (DHT); 99% is bound and only 1% is free and available for conversion.

Derangements in the biosynthesis and metabolism of endocrine substances can have lasting effects in either sex, for in every individual the glands of internal secretion significantly affect the activity of every cell in the body. It is the function of the endocrine glands, such as the pituitary, the thyroid, adrenals, reproductive organs (testes and ovaries) and others to maintain the constancy of the body's chemistry. Therefore, a survey of the endocrine glands, their bodily function, and relationships to hair growth, is important to any discussion of abnormal hair growth (Figure 5 and 6).

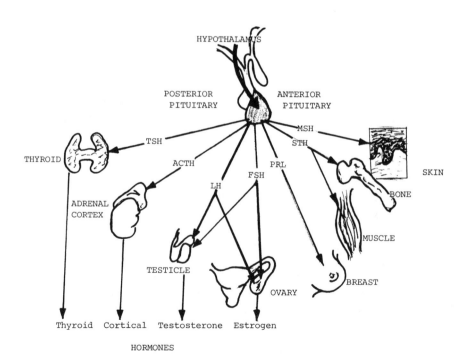

Figure 5. Endocrine glands and hormones.

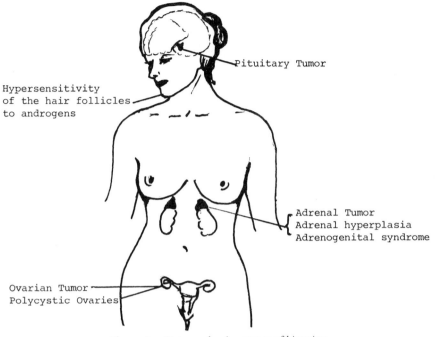

Pituitary Tumor

Hypersensitivity
of the hair follicles
to androgens

Adrenal Tumor
Adrenal hyperplasia
Adrenogenital syndrome

Ovarian Tumor
Polycystic Ovaries

Figure 6.   Major endocrine causes of hirsutism.

THE ENDOCRINE GLANDS

The endocrine glands are the same in men and women, except for their respective reproductive organs. These glands secrete hormones into the blood stream to form a chemical system of communication between cells and also collaborate with the nervous system via the hypothalamus to adjust the body to internal and external buffetings of the environment. Under rare circumstances too much or too little of these specific compounds may be manufactured, resulting in certain disease states.

The hypothalamic-pituitary axis

The hypothalamus is part of the midbrain, the diencephalon, and provides the connective link between the cerebral cortex of the brain and the pituitary gland. Certain metabolic functions under the control of the hypothalamus are of considerable importance to the endocrine system because stimulatory and inhibitory agents that originate in the hypothalamus influence pituitary function.

Before man evolved to his present station, it is believed that the original brain was not covered by the cortex (outer brain). In primitive man, the hypothalamus was the 'old brain', where instincts necessary to preserve the species originated, such as procreation, flight from danger, and fight for self preservation. With the acquisition of a cortex, man acquired intellect, memory, thought processes and rationalization.

The hypothalamus is intimately concerned with regulation of the body's energy balance through control of appetite, sleep, body temperature, regulation of sexual function and control of water balance. Lesions or disturbances in the hypothalamus may cause such endocrine disorders as sexual precocity or sexual infantilism; absence of appetite with extreme weight loss, or insatiable appetite with enormous obesity; diabetes insipidus with excessive thirst and uncontrollable output of large amounts of urine; disorganization of sleep rhythms, as well as hibernating (low) and extremely high body temperatures. Because the hypothalamus is part of the central nervous system, emotional disturbances, anxiety, worry, or aberrations in thought processes of the brain may upset hypothalamic-pituitary mechanisms and result in abnormal hair growth.

Hypertrichosis has been observed in children following concussion of the brain and encephalitis (infection of the brain). Patients with anorexia nervosa, a severe disorder of the neuroendocrine system characterized by voluntary starvation and loss of menstrual periods, frequently develop fine dark hair on the face, trunk and arms. An increase in body hair growth can also occur in severe involuntary starvation or chronic illness. Some women have developed increased hair growth following severe psychogenic stress, and women institutionalized in mental hospitals are frequently more hirsute than nonpsychotic women.

The pituitary gland, also called the hypophysis, is a small round structure, 13 mm in diameter and weighing 0.6 g, situated at the base of the skull in a small deep cavity known as the sella turcica (Turk's saddle). It is attached to the brain by a thin stalk, and is divided into an anterior portion, composed of glandular tissue, and a posterior portion, composed of nerve-like tissue, which is an extension of the hypothalamus, that portion of the brain to which the pituitary stalk is attached. Both parts of the gland produce a number of hormones under hypothalamic control which influence or stimulate distant structures or target glands.

The target glands for the hormones produced by the anterior pituitary are the thyroid, adrenal cortex, the testes and ovaries. The other endocrine glands are not directly influenced by the pituitary. A discussion of each of the hormones, their bodily function and relationship, if any, to hair growth follows:

1. *Growth stimulating hormone* is essential for growth, not only of cartilage and bone, but other bodily tissues as well, and is thought to influence genetic hair growth. If the secretion of this hormone is insufficient during the formative years, or if the pituitary gland is removed during that period of

development, statural growth is limited and dwarfism results. Excessive production of the hormone in adults causes acromegaly, i.e., gross enlargement of the face, hands, feet, and internal organs. Female acromegalics may manifest hirsutism.

2. *Adrenocorticotrophin (ACTH)* stimulates the adrenal cortex: too little ACTH atrophies the cortical layers of the gland; too much causes the cortex to enlarge (hypertrophy). Our ability to withstand prolonged periods of stress depends on the ability of the pituitary gland to respond to such situations by adequate secretion of ACTH to stimulate the adrenal glands. Increased stimulation results in increased production of androgens by the adrenal, thus an increase in hair growth.

3. *Thyroid stimulating hormone (TSH),* as the name suggests, stimulates the thyroid gland to produce hormones which regulate the body's metabolism.

4. *Gonadotrophins* stimulate the reproductive organs, i.e., testes and ovaries. In both sexes the gonadotrophins are a follicle stimulating hormone (FSH) and a luteinizing hormone (LH). In the male, LH is also known as ICSH (interstitial cell-stimulating hormone), and in both sexes LH stimulates androgen production by the respective gonads. In the female, increased LH secretion results in ovarian stromal hyperactivity, thus hyperandrogenism and the development of hirsutism.

5. *Prolactin (PRL)* stimulates breast milk production. Breastfeeding or suckling stimulates the pituitary to produce prolactin. Too much of this hormone results in the syndrome of persistent lactation in non-pregnant women, as well as amenorrhea (absence of menses) and infertility. Increased prolactin production may also stimulate adrenal androgen production and thus the development of excess hair growth.

6. *Melanocyte stimulating hormone (MSH)* brings about darkening of the skin, especially after exposure to sunlight. Light regulates the secretion of MSH via the hypothalamus. Its secretion accounts for the characteristic pigmentation associated with various disorders, such as Addison's disease, which is chronic adrenal insufficiency. During pregnancy, MSH activity may produce the abnormal pigmentation of the face known as the 'mask of pregnancy'.

The posterior portion of the pituitary gland stores and secretes two hormones: (1) *vasopressin,* the antidiuretic hormone (ADH), influences renal duct permeability and water metabolism. In high concentrations it also causes contraction of the smooth muscle in blood vessels, thus causing high blood pressure. Alcohol consumption decreases ADH secretion and results in the increased urine production so typically associated with alcohol ingestion. The other hormone produced is (2) *oxytocin.* The secretion of oxytocin causes vigorous contractions of the uterus during labor, as well as the contraction of muscle cells lining breast ducts to aid in the flow of milk after birth of a baby.

The pineal gland

The pineal gland is situated at the base of the brain and is shaped like a pine cone. Until recently little was known of the function of this gland and it was believed to be merely a vestigial organ that may have once served a purpose in the course of human development. Early anatomy studies postulated a relationship between the pineal gland and the possession of a thin skin, because it was noted that in thick-skinned animal species the pineal was absent, but was well developed in those with a relatively thin skin.[4] A connection between the pineal and the reproductive system was first discovered in 1898, when it was found that a tumor of the pineal gland caused sexual precocity in a $4\frac{1}{2}$ year old male child; other cases have also been reported.[5] Recent studies have shown that the pineal has stimulatory and inhibitory influences on the hypothalamus and researchers have begun to investigate the connection between the pineal and the effects of light on reproductive cycles. The role of the pineal remains uncertain, but it is believed to be that of fine adjustment of reproductive processes and other homeostatic mechanisms that help the body adapt to changes in environment.[6]

The thyroid gland

The thyroid gland is the central organ in a system that incorporates iodine into compounds of hormonal activity, and makes them available for action in bodily tissues. The thyroid is composed of two lobes joined by an isthmus, or constricted part, and weighs about an ounce or less. It lies in front of and on either side of the windpipe just beneath the larynx, or voice-box. Proper function of the thyroid gland is dependent on normal pituitary function and upon a sufficient supply of iodine from food and water. Iodine, combined with certain amino acids, is stored as thyroglobulin and is released from the thyroid gland into the blood stream in the form of thyroxine, which affects the body's metabolism and is required for normal growth and development of the brain, the muscles and bones. Too much thyroid leads to hyperthyroidism with symptoms of apprehension, nervousness, loss of weight, increased thirst, frequent urination, profuse perspiration, intolerance of heat, insomnia, frequent stools, rapid heart beat and palpitations. Too little thyroid hormone produces a low metabolic rate and slows down all the body's biologic processes. Inadequate iodine supplies and excessive intake of iodides or certain drugs that impede hormone synthesis may result in thyroid enlargement and goiter development.

Hyperthyroidism does not cause excessive hair growth; however juvenile hypothyroidism has been implicated as a cause of hypertrichosis. This is due to a deficiency of thyroid hormone which results in a decrease in SHBG and an increase in free testosterone levels. The hair growth is the long lanugo type.

The parathyroid glands

There are four parathyroid glands, and each is only slightly larger than a small bead. They are superficially imbedded on the back and side surfaces of each lobe of the thyroid gland. These glands produce two hormones, *parathormone* and *calcitonin,* whose function is to maintain a stable concentration of calcium in the blood. Parathormone is released whenever blood calcium levels are low to activate the transfer of calcium from bone to blood until calcium levels return to normal. Calcitonin is released during periods of excess calcium in the blood. Excessive hormone production causes serious bone disorders or kidney stones, and decreased production leads to neuromuscular excitability. Hypoparathyroidism causes hair to become sparse, dry and brittle due to decreased calcium levels which affect hair development at the cellular level.

The thymus gland

The thymus lies high in the chest. It is relatively large in infants but is greatly diminished in size in adults and is thought to play a role in inciting immunological processes that give resistance to disease and infections. There is no known connection to hair growth.

The pancreas gland

The pancreas is located in the abdomen and has both an endocrine and an exocrine portion. The exocrine function is to secrete digestive juices into the upper intestinal tract. The endocrine portion consists of alpha and beta cells lying in small clusters which are known as the islets of Langerhans. The beta cells produce insulin; the alpha cells produce glucagon. Glucagon raises blood sugar levels while insulin reduces them. Insulin is, therefore, essential for proper metabolism of glucose. An insufficient production of insulin results in diabetes, a condition in which blood sugar levels rise markedly. Hypoglycemia develops when blood sugar levels decline. A possible relationship between diabetes and hirsutism is discussed in Chapter 6.

The adrenal glands

The adrenals are two small, triangular-shaped glands lying immediately in front of and above each kidney. Each gland consists of a medulla and a cortex. Both play important roles in health and disease.

The medulla is intimately connected to the sympathetic nervous system and its hormones are *epinephrine* (adrenalin) and *norepinephrine* (noradrenalin). Adrenalin is vital in enabling an individual to meet sudden dangers and emergencies and prepares the way for quick action. Adrenalin and noradrenalin secretion is triggered by the alarm reaction and summons reserve strength for flight or fight, and, if wounded, to minimize blood loss through constriction of blood vessels and faster clotting time. Epinephrine stimulates the pituitary to produce more ACTH hormone, which in turn increases adrenal cortex function. The adrenal releases glucocorticoids to induce conversion of glucose from proteins and replenish sugar stores in the liver and muscle that were used up in the alarm reaction. Occasionally, tumors that secrete an excess amount of epinephrine and/or norepinephrine may arise in the medulla of one or both glands. Excess epinephrine production causes apprehension, tremor, palpitations, sweating, headache, abdominal cramps, nausea and vomiting. Excess norepinephrine production causes a marked and sustained rise in blood pressure. The most striking symptoms are paroxysmal attacks of high blood pressure which may later develop into a chronic blood pressure elevation.

The adrenal cortex secretes three types of hormones: (1) *glucocorticoids* that influence carbohydrate, protein and fat metabolism; (2) *mineralocorticoids* that regulate salt and water balances; and (3) *steroid hormones* that act as an auxiliary source of male and female sex hormones. Excessive steroid hormone secretion by the adrenals may be due to either stress, hyperplasia, or a tumor. The main sex steroids produced in cases of hyperplasia are androgens, which produce virilism (masculinity) and hirsutism in the female and precocious puberty in the male. A tumor, on the other hand, produces either androgens or estrogens in a paradoxical manner. As a result, the female is masculinized while the male is feminized by the excess steroid secretion. The disorders associated with adrenal cortical dysfunction are discussed in detail in other chapters of this book.

The male and female reproductive organs (gonads)

The testicles or male gonads lie in the scrotal sac; the normal size varies from that of a walnut to that of a pigeon egg. The function of these glands is the production and excretion of sperm by the tubules and the production of *testosterone,* the principal androgen in the male. The testes also produce small amounts of estrogens. At puberty, testosterone production increases and induces maturation of the secondary sex characteristics, i.e., full development of the penis, increased muscle mass, voice changes, pubic and axillary hair growth, and eventual beard and body hair growth.

The ovaries of the female also have two functions: one is to provide ova (egg cells) necessary for conception, and the other is to produce sex hormones. The ovaries are awakened to activity at puberty, which usually begins between ages 11 and 13. The major hormones produced by the ovary are *estrogens* and *progesterone,* but small quantities of *androgens* are also produced. These hormones serve to develop the secondary female sex characteristics, i.e., breast growth, maturation of the genital tract, pubic and axillary hair growth, as well as the graceful contours of the female body. During the reproductive years, there is a cyclic production of estrogen followed by estrogen and progesterone. If an ovum is fertilized and it is then implanted in the hormonally prepared endometrium (lining of the uterus), a fetus will grow. The placenta, the special structure that develops from the implanted embryo and which later becomes the afterbirth, also produces hormones necessary to support and maintain the pregnancy. If conception does not occur, ovarian hormone production ceases toward the end of each cycle, and hormonal support to the endometrium is withdrawn. Shedding of the lining takes place with the passage of blood, hence the monthly period.

Inadequate or absent ovarian stimulation by the pituitary gonadotropic hormones, failure of the ovary to respond, or an abnormal response to hormone stimulation, results in many menstrual disorders during the reproductive years, which range from complete failure to menstruate (amenorrhea), to excessive flow (hypermenorrhea). An ovarian increase in androgen production may result from either enzymatic blocks at the ovary, hypothalamic estrogen insensitivity, or from increased LH secretion by the pituitary which results in ovarian stromal hyperactivity and increased hair growth.

As a woman ages, reproductive function comes to an end, and she enters the menopause, which means cessation of menses. Coincident with the loss of reproductive capacity, there is a decline in hormone production by the ovaries. With the decrease in estrogen levels there is an increase in the amount of free testosterone available for conversion to DHT. Many menopausal women experience unwanted hair growth, as well as varying degrees of vasomotor instability, i.e., hot flushes, night sweats, depression, headaches, bladder irritations, urinary incontinence, senile vaginitis, as well as demineralization of bone (osteoporosis) and joint aches.

WHEN IS A HORMONE PROFILE NECESSARY?

The physician to whom a hirsute woman turns for help must first determine the cause of the disorder because not all cases of unwanted hair are due to an endocrine dysfunction. The majority of hirsute women have the primary type due to increased follicle sensitivity or genetic predisposition. There are striking differences among the various races in distribution of hair, rate of growth, and type of hair. Caucasians have a greater number of hair follicles as compared to Orientals, American Indians, or Blacks, and Caucasians of peri-Mediterranean regions are frequently more hairy than their northern European cousins. In multinational, outbred populations, such as exists in the

United States, there are multifold differences in genetic potential for hair growth as well.[7] In addition, central nervous system mechanisms may also alter rates of production or degradation of androgens or alter hair follicle activity by nervous stimulation or by increased blood flow.[7] Both stress and emotional instability influence hair growth, as does aging and certain drugs.

Therefore, to rule out a systemic endocrine disorder of either adrenal or ovarian origin, it is essential for the physician to first ascertain racial origins, familial history, duration and sites of hair growth, and mode of progression. If hyperandrogenism is suspected, he also needs to learn what signs and symptoms are associated with the onset of abnormal growth, such as menstrual disorders, voice changes, enlargement of the clitoris, increases in muscle mass and strength, as well as what medications have been administered, or if there is a history of repeated psychic trauma. A thorough personal history of past illnesses, including pregnancies, abortions, and miscarriages is also essential. Only after such evaluation will he/she be able to determine which patient fits the primary or idiopathic type and which has a possible endocrine disorder and needs to undergo hormonal evaluation to establish and treat the cause.

Ongoing research has allowed great strides to be made thus far in the diagnosis and treatment of the various endocrinopathies. When an endocrine disorder is suspected, the physician has at his/her disposal several laboratory evaluations that aid in diagnosing the cause. The development of radioimmunoassay (RIA) has enabled the sensitive measurement of androgens, even in minute quantities, in the blood. Radioactive isotopes have helped in the understanding of the metabolism of these hormones; catheterization of adrenal and ovarian veins to obtain selective venous effluents has helped to determine the origin of these androgens.

(a)   Serum testosterone: A level of less than 2 ng/ml will rule out testosterone secreting tumors of the ovary or adrenal (normal = 0.2-0.8 ng/ml). A level greater than 2 ng/ml requires that further ovarian and adrenal evaluation be undertaken.

(b)   Serum DHEA-S or 17-ketosteroids are measured in 24 hour urines for evaluation of androgen excess from the adrenal glands. If there is a suspicion of cortisol excess, an overnight dexamethasone suppression is done. Serum cortisol is measured at 8 a.m. and the patient is given 1 mg of dexamethasone at 11 p.m.; serum cortisol is again measured the next morning at 8 a.m. If the cortisol level is greater than 5 ng/dl, a 5-day dexamethasone suppression test should be done to rule out adrenal tumor. These tumors have high DHEA-S levels and are not suppressed by high doses of dexamethasone. Computerized axial tomography (CAT scan) is also employed to diagnose these tumors.

(c)   ACTH: Radioimmunoassay of adrenocorticotropic hormone (ACTH) is helpful in evaluating some cases of adrenocortical dysfunction.

Low levels point to adrenal disease and high levels indicate pituitary disease or other ectopic ACTH producing tumors.

(d) Prolactin (PRL) levels should be measured; if they are high, prolactin secreting pituitary adenomas should be ruled out because some cases of polycystic ovaries (Stein-Leventhal Syndrome) have elevated PRL levels with pituitary microadenomas.[8] DHEA and DHEA-S are increased in hyperprolactinemia. The percentage of amenorrheic women with hirsutism increases in the presence of a high prolactin level.

(e) Serum thyroid stimulating hormone (TSH), thyroxine (T4) and triiodothyronine (T3) should be measured because protracted treatment of hypothyroid conditions leads to an increase of plasma DHEA and DHEA-S.

(f) Free Steroids (testosterone glucuronide, DHT, and 3α – and 3β – androstanediol) should also be measured because they provide a suitable screening test to demonstrate whether hyperandrogenism is present or not.

SUMMARY

Before the entry of endocrinology as a full fledged discipline into the field of medicine, little was known or understood of the chemical system of communication between cells that enables mankind to adjust to the changing environment, heat and cold, food excesses and deprivations, the stresses of injury, infection and emotional strain. Most cases of pituitary dwarfism or giantism, severe anorexia or obesity, as well as hirsute or virilized women, were relegated by society into the realm of the side show or circus as 'freaks'. Through ongoing research and the ever increasing knowledge of basic physiologic, pathologic, biochemical and genetic principles, the importance of the endocrine system and of the hormonal imbalances that adversely affect the way we think and behave, our physical agility, build and stature, voice pitch, sexual urge, reproductive capacity, and hair growth, are better understood.

Understanding is also by necessity the first step in successful treatment of any disorder, but is especially so in cases of hirsutism. Unwanted hair growth in a female of any age – child, teenager, or adult – is emotionally devastating. Stress and emotional factors can increase excessive hair growth in either primary or secondary hirsutism, making them all the more difficult for the physician to manage. The physician must understand that in addition to the newer methods available for diagnosis and treatment, the patient needs a great deal of psychological support as well to reduce emotional stress. The patient must understand that even though the physician can provide treatment to prevent new hair growth and correct endocrine disorders, established hairs did not develop overnight and will not go away rapidly.

Because of the knowledge gained over the past few decades, both idiopathic and true hirsutism can now be successfully managed, and the physician no longer needs to suffer frustration in his/her attempts to treat a hirsute patient because of having little else to offer except sympathy and to suggest that she shave, tweeze, or use depilatory agents. However, the greatest benefit of all is the fact that the hirsute female no longer needs to fear the loss of her essential femininity and reproductive capacity, or to long endure the curiosity and possible ridicule of society. Medical treatment will correct endocrine disorders and prevent the development of new hair growth; electrolysis will permanently remove unwanted hair.

References

1. Segre, E. J., *Androgens, Virilization and the Hirsute Female*. Springfield, Charles C. Thomas, 1967
2. Breuer, H., Androgen production in women. In, *Androgens in Women: Acne, Seborrhoea, Androgenic Alopecia and Hirsutism*. Hammerstein, L., Lachnit-Fixon, U., Neumann, F. and Plewig, G., (eds). Amsterdam, Excerpta Medica, 1980, pp 21-39
3. *Gray's Anatomy, Descriptive and Applied*. Howden, R., (ed). Toronto, Longmans, Green and Co, Ltd., 1926, p 852
4. Janne, O. A. and Bardin C. W., Mechanisms of action of androgens and antiandrogens. In, *Hirsutism and Virilism: Pathogenesis, Diagnosis and Management*. Mahesh, V. B. and Greenblatt. R. B. (eds). Boston, Bristol, London, John Wright PSG, 1983, p 283
5. Selye, H., The Pineal. In, *Textbook of Endocrinology*. Montreal, Acta Endocrinologica, 1947, pp 593-599
6. Hoffman, J. C., The influence of photoperiods on reproductive function in female animals. *Handbook of Physiology, Sect. 7: Endocrinology, Vol. II*. Greep, R. O. and Astwood, E. B., (eds). Washington, D. C., American Physiol Soc, 1973, pp 57-77
7. Hamilton, J. B., Racial and genetic predisposition. In, *The Hirsute Female*. Hughes E. C., (ed). Clin Obstet Gynecol 7:1075, 1964
8. Tzingounis, V., Alperin, H. and Natrajan, P. K., Radiographic abnormalities in patients with Stein-Leventhal syndrome. Int J Gynecol Obstet 16:166, 1978

5
Iatrogenic Hirsutism

Anthony E. Karpas, M.D.

Iatrogenic hirsutism and hypertrichosis are extremely distressing side effects of a small group of drugs in a minority of treated patients. The term iatrogenic denotes a drug-induced or physician caused condition. While both forms of unwanted hair growth are not life-threatening, they can be psychologically very damaging, especially in children and adolescent girls. Because there are effective substitutes for almost all of the drugs responsible, careful monitoring and timely action should prevent increased hair growth in the majority of cases.

Medications which have the ability to induce abnormal or excessive hair growth can be divided into two groups according to the pattern of hair growth and the presumed cause. The first group consists of hormonal drugs with androgenic properties which cause growth on areas of the body normally associated with male secondary sexual distribution. This pattern of hair growth is referred to as hirsutism. The hair is of the coarse terminal type and grows on the beard and moustache areas of the face, on the chest, around the nipples, below the umbilicus, and on the back. The second group of drugs are nonhormonal, and cause a different pattern of hair growth which is generally referred to as hypertrichosis. The hair is finer and is midway in thickness between vellus and terminal hair. Hair growth appears on the face, temples, and forehead above and beside the eyebrows. Hairs on the back of the arms lengthen and increase in number, and the lower legs and trunk are also usually affected. Typically, the axilla and pubic areas are spared. This type of drug-induced hair growth is more common in children and is generally, but not invariably, reversible within a few months after cessation of the medication.

ANDROGENIC HAIR GROWTH, OR HIRSUTISM

Hirsutism or androgen-stimulated hair growth is, as mentioned elsewhere in this book, the result of stimulation of those hair follicles carrying androgen receptors. Conversion of testosterone to dihydrotestosterone (DHT) by the skin is believed to be necessary. By increasing testosterone from its binding protein, or by interfering in its metabolism, the amount of free testosterone available for conversion to DHT would be increased. Some drugs may act by direct stimulation of receptors of the androgen sensitive hair follicle.

Individual women vary greatly in their sensitivity to androgens, with brunettes of Mediterranean extraction allegedly being most sensitive, probably due to an increased efficiency of conversion of testosterone to DHT in the skin. Most of the androgenic medications mentioned below tend to cause hirsutism only in sensitive individuals.

Testosterone

In sufficient quantities, testosterone will invariably cause hirsutism in women. The use of low doses of testosterone in conjunction with estrogen therapy to increase anabolic activity, libido, and well being has been advocated in treatment of the menopause.[1] It is also used to treat aplastic anemias, as well as women with breast cancer. However, women treated with testosterone should always be monitored for the presence of virilizing side effects, and if acne or hirsutism appear, the dose, where possible, should be decreased or the drug discontinued.

Danazol

Danazol is an attenuated androgen used in the treatment of endometriosis, cystic breast conditions, and angioneurotic edema. The use of danazol has been associated with a 5.5% incidence of a mild degree of hirsutism in one series and 5.8% in another,[2,3] and is reported to occur mainly in brunettes with a tendency to oily skin. Other signs of androgen action, such as acne and voice changes, have also been reported, while clitoral enlargement is an occasional complication.

Danazol has been found to have weak androgen action in castrated rats and may directly interact with the androgen receptor to cause increased hair growth. Another explanation may be a lowering of the estrogen levels due to danazol's gonadotropin suppressing effects, thus changing the estrogen: androgen ratio. The lower estrogen levels would also cause the level of the sex hormone binding globulin (SHBG) to decrease. In addition, danazol may also displace testosterone from its binding globulin, with the net result being more free testosterone for conversion to dihydrotestosterone (DHT). Most of the androgenic actions of danazol have only been found at the highest dose of 800 mg per day; reduction of the dosage to 400 mg or less per day may prevent further problems without losing the beneficial effects of therapy.

Oral contraceptives

Hirsutism is listed as a side effect of oral contraceptives in the Physician's Desk Reference (PDR) and in the drug company literature provided for the patient. While this is more theoretical than real, there are potential causes. Norgestrel and norethindrone are two of the progestational agents commonly used in combination oral birth control pills. They have some mild androgenic properties and norethindrone has been shown to have 2% of the androgenic potency of testosterone. The anabolic potency is estimated at 10%. The reason hirsutism does not occur with birth control pills is because the estrogens in the pill over-ride the weak androgenic activity of these progestogens derived from testosterone. In fact, oral contraceptives are very effective in treating hirsutism, as discussed more completely in Chapter 10.

D-Norgestrel has been shown to decrease the binding of testosterone to SHBG, and also to displace testosterone from SHBG, thus increasing free testosterone levels. While the estrogen in oral contraceptives raises SHBG levels and usually offsets this effect, the use of increasingly lower doses of estrogen in contraceptives, and the use of progesterone only contraceptives, may theoretically be associated with some excessive hair growth; however, in actual practice this has not been a problem, probably because of the lowered dosages of progestogens. Women experiencing acne or hirsutism, or thought to be at increased risk for these problems, should be advised to use an estrogen dominant birth control pill (see Chapter 10).

Synthetic glucocorticoids

Hirsutism is a rare complication of synthetic glucocorticoids (adrenal-like hormones) administration. A case has been reported of florid Cushing's syndrome and hirsutism following absorption of topical dexamethasone (DXS) in a patient with extensive skin lesions due to psoriasis. The hirsutism could be attributed to the loss of the C_{21} side chain, resulting in the formation of 17-ketosteroid components. Since these compounds tend to be androgenic, this probably is responsible for the patient's hirsutism.

Adrenocorticotrophin (ACTH)

Synthetic ACTH compounds (adrenal-stimulating hormones) have been used therapeutically in order to treat steroid-sensitive conditions without causing adrenal suppression. Such treatment would also stimulate adrenal androgens and could result in excess hair growth. This is also more theoretical than factual.

Metyrapone

Metyrapone (an adrenal hormone antagonist) has been advocated as an alternative to adrenalectomy in the long-term management of Cushing's disease when due to hyperplasia rather than a tumor. Virilization as a result of accumulation of 11-deoxycorticoids and androgens could occur. In one study, hirsutism was noted in five of seven women treated: one patient had exceptionally high testosterone levels (16 ng/ml) and had to have an adrenalectomy due to unacceptable virilization. In two others, testosterone levels were in excess of 100 ng/ml.[4]

Phenothiazine

Phenothiazines (tranquilizers) used in psychiatric practice are known to stimulate prolactin production, thus interfering with normal estrogen secretion; but the mechanism of action is unclear. A case of hirsutism induced by phenothiazine therapy in a chronically schizophrenic patient has been reported.[5] However, stress, which is also associated with hirsutism, may have been a factor in this particular case.

Anabolic Steroids

Anabolic steroids are being increasingly used by women preoccupied with athletic performance. Some of these are structurally related to androgens, and hirsutism could be a complication of such compounds.

DRUGS CAUSING HYPERTRICHOSIS

Drugs that cause hypertrichosis probably do not alter any known hormonal mechanism. No increase in testosterone, DHT, androstenedione, 17-ketosteroids, or 17-hydroxysteroids has been reported in association with this type of hair growth. The mechanism of action is unknown and may vary depending on the offending drug employed. This complication is much more common in children than in adults; however, hypertrichosis, once established, has not been reported to lessen with puberty. Removing the offending drug may result in remission.

Phenytoin

Phenytoin (Dilantin), used to treat epilepsy, is probably the drug most commonly associated with hypertrichosis. The first association was described in 1955, and others have reported it to occur in 5% to 12% of patients treated.[6] Hypertrichosis generally appears two to three months after the onset of therapy and most of the growth appears on the extremities; however, some growth is noted on the trunk as well. A few patients have profuse growth of moustache hair, but the pubes and axilla are spared in prepubertal children, which suggests that the mechanism of action is non-androgenic. Why the hair growth is more pronounced on the uncovered or sun exposed areas is unknown. Although improvement may occur on discontinuation of the drug, hair growth is generally irreversible.

The appearance of hypertrichosis is not correlated with dose of serum Dilantin levels, and it is postulated that the enlargement of hairs is primarily due to the enlargement of all elements of the connective tissue, including the hair papilla. Supporting this is the fact that the added tissue in gingival hyperplasia, which is associated with hirsutism, is primarily a result of hyperplasia of submucosal connective tissue (Figs 1 and 2).[7]

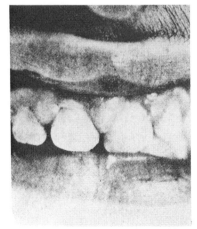

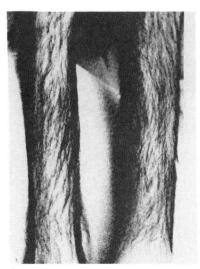

Figure 1. Gingival hyperplasia and hirsute upper lip, secondary to Dilantin, in a 22-year-old woman. (Reproduced from Van Scott E. J., Clin Obstet Gynecol 7:1062, 1964)

Figure 2. Lower legs of same patient. Note abundant hair growth (From: IBID)

Diazoxide

Diazoxide is an anti-insulin and antihypertensive drug used in the treatment of hypoglycemia (low blood sugar levels) in children. In adults diazoxide is used to treat acute malignant hypertension and chronic hypertensive kidney disease. In eight children treated for hypoglycemia, hair growth occurred within six weeks after treatment was begun and affected the forehead, sideburns, nape of the neck, and the back of the trunk and extremities.[8] Hair thickness was intermediate and no sexual hair growth was seen. Biopsy showed many hair follicles to be in the anagen growth cycle, with large amounts of glycogen and a rich vascular network. No increases in sebaceous glands were seen however, which ruled out androgen effects.

Hypertrichosis in treated adults probably occurs in less than 1%, and complete remission of hirsutism occurs on discontinuation of the medication. Increased cutaneous perfusion has been postulated to be the cause of the hair growth, since it is occasionally seen overlying arteriovenous aneurysms (weakness in blood vessel walls) and in association with inflammation. This effect is not seen in other drugs with a similar mode of action, nor is it seen with psoriasis which causes cutaneous hyperemia (increased blood to the skin). Another possible explanation was a direct pharmacological effect on the hair follicle.

Minoxidil

Minoxidil is a newly released drug used in the treatment of malignant hypertension, a rapidly progressive form of high blood pressure that is often fatal. The use of minoxidil in patients with severe kidney disease can be life-saving, but the excess hair growth can be an extremely distressing side effect. The hypertrichosis seen with minoxidil has been compared to that seen with diazoxide, but the difference in incidence between the two drugs would seem to argue against an identical mechanism of action.

In a study of 87 patients, hypertrichosis was a universal complaint.[9] Hair distribution was widespread, but was more prominent on the arms and face, and facial hair was associated with a coarsening of facial features. The condition was of a severe enough nature to cause three women to cease further therapy.

Earhart et al, reporting on the use of calcium thioglycolate depilatories, found that while they were less effective than barium sulfide in removing terminal hair, they were also less irritating.[10] Since the hair seen with minoxidil is of the thinner nonterminal type, calcium thioglycolate produced excellent cosmetic results and minimal irritation. Thus, hirsutism should not be a reason to withhold minoxidil therapy.

Adrenal hormones

High-dose glucocorticoids (Cortisone) given for long periods of time are occasionally associated with hypertrichosis. This hair growth is not of the androgenic variety seen with Cushing's disease and is probably due to the conversion of telogen to anagen hair by these adrenal hormones. Local injections of these drugs can cause a remission of the patches of hair loss seen with alopecia areata (spotty baldness). However, this effect may be due to a decrease in the action of autoantibodies on the affected hair follicles. A decrease in the clearance of prednisolone may be responsible in patients with side effects of prednisone therapy, including hirsutism and a change in fat distribution. Efficacy of therapy was also related to decreased clearance.

Hexachlorobenzine

In 1955, a sudden and devastating outbreak of an unusual type of skin disorder (porphyria cutanea tarda) occurred in Turkey. A fungicide, hexachlorobenzine, had been added to wheat prepared for planting. Contrary to intent, this wheat was consumed by the local peasant populace. Three thousand cases of porphyria, a disease causing dark urine and serious problems, were reported with extreme photosensitivity of the skin pigmentation and hirsutism of a much greater degree than is usually encountered with other types of porphyria (Figs. 3 and 4). The face, extremities, and whole body were covered with hair. The unusual pigmentation and hirsutism gave these children a simian appearance, and they were referred to as 'monkey children' by the local inhabitants. No abdominal symptoms or neurologic (nerve) disorders are associated with this type of porphyria; however, liver enlargement and severe impairment of liver function were seen. Large quantities of porphyrin were found in the urine but not in the feces. Most patients recovered, with the urine returning to normal 30 days after discontinuing ingestion of the poisoned wheat. In some cases, however, relapses occurred during the summer, while in others acute symptoms persisted.

Streptomycin

Streptomycin (a potent antibiotic) was reported to cause hypertrichosis in children being treated for tuberculosis,[11, 12] and has long been listed as a side effect of this therapy. However, such children are usually debilitated and increased hair growth has been found in association with debilitation. Furthermore, hypertrichosis has been found in children with tuberculosis but not on streptomycin therapy.

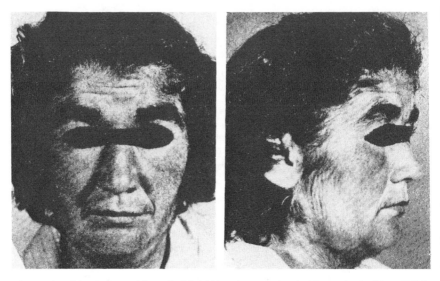

Figures 3 and 4. Patient with marked facial hirsutism associated with porphyria. (From IBID)

Penicillamine

Penicillamine, used as a chelator and in the treatment of refractory rheumatoid arthritis, causes thickening and coarsening of the hair on the trunk and limbs.

Psoralens

Instances of hair growth on the vitilingenous area of the body or on parts exposed to the sun have been found after use of methoxypsoralen. The local redness and thickening of the skin in the areas of sun exposure after psoralen therapy were thought responsible.

CONCLUSION

As man evolved toward an erect posture, he also lost his furry hair covering. In today's society, hair on women is considered to detract from femininity. Daily TV commercials for a variety of feminine shaving devices, waxes, and depilatories reinforce the belief, and the appearance of hair on areas of the body where such growth is not usual is, therefore, regarded with much alarm.

Drugs working via androgenic mechanisms should be avoided in women with a predisposition to hirsutism. In cases where excessive growth is the presenting complaint, a drug history is mandatory. As has been mentioned, there are effective substitutes for almost all of the drugs discussed in this chapter. An awareness of the problem and adequate monitoring of the patient should allow early adjustment of therapy and thereby avoid subsequent patient anxiety.

Hypertrichosis also causes much distress, as it occurs most commonly in prepubertal girls and persists throughout puberty. It is generally less of a problem to deal with than hirsutism, as the hair is thinner and easier to remove. However, facial hair growth may cause enough anxiety to cause the patient to demand discontinuing the drug. Where the drug is considered indispensable to treatment, the patient can be assured that shaving does not cause hair to thicken, and the use of bleaches, depilatories and plucking are also effective though only temporary measures. Electrolysis should be recommended for permanent removal of the unwanted hair.

References

1. Greenblatt, R. B., Nezhat, C. and Karpas, A. The menopausal syndrome: hormone replacement therapy. In, *The Menopause: Comprehensive Management,* Eskin B.A. (ed). New York, Masson, 1980, p 151
2. Young, M. D. and Blackmore, W. P. The use of danazol in the management of endometriosis. J Int Med Res 5:86, 1977
3. Rakoff, A. E. Side effects of danazol therapy. In, *Recent Advances in Endometriosis.* Excerpta Medica Internat Congr Series 368, 1976, p 108
4. Jeffcoate, W. J., Rees, L. H. and Tomlin S, et al: Metyrapone in long-term management of Cushing's disease. Br Med J 2:215, 1977
5. Phillips, P., Shraberg, D. and Weitzel, W. D. Hirsutism associated with long-term phenothiazine neuroleptic therapy. JAMA 241:920, 1979
6. Livingston, S., Petersen, D. and Boks L. L. Medical treatment of Epilepsy: "Dilantin". In, *Comprehensive Management of Epilepsy in Infancy, Childhood and Adolescence.* Springfield, IL., Charles C. Thomas, 1972, p 189
7. Van Scott, E. J. The hirsute female: Physiology of hair growth. Clin Obstet Gynecol 7:1062, 1964
8. Baker, L., Kaye, R. and Root, A. W., et al: Diazoxide treatment of idiopathic hypoglycemia of infancy. J Pediatr 71:449, 1967
9. Mackay, A., Henderson I. and Fife, R., et al: Minoxidil in the management of interactable hypertension. Q J Med 198: 175, 1981
10. Earhart, R. N., Ball, J. and Nuss, D. D., et al: Minoxidil induced hypertrichosis: Treatment with calcium thioglycolate depilatory. South Med J 70:442, 1977
11. Muller, S. A. Hirsutism. Am J Med 46:803, 1969
12. Fono, R. Appearance of hypertrichosis during streptomycin treatment. Ann Pediatr 174:389, 1950

6
Unusual Syndromes
A. Diabetes of the Bearded Woman (Achard-Thiers)
B. Acanthosis Nigricans

Robert B. Greenblatt, M.D.

DIABETES OF THE BEARDED WOMAN

Achard and Thiers in 1921 reported a case of a 71-year-old woman with hirsutism and transitory glycosuria (sugar in the urine) in whom autopsy revealed enlarged adrenal glands and other minor pathological findings in the pancreas and thyroid gland.[1] They believed this condition was due to a pluriglandular defect and called it "Diabète des femmes à barbe" (the diabetes of bearded women). The clinical association of glycosuria and hirsutism, sometimes along with obesity and hypertension had been reported previously by Kraus and by Tuffler.[2,3] In 1932, Cushing reported 14 cases in whom the cardinal symptoms were obesity, hirsutism, diabetes and hypertension.[4] Most of these patients were shown to have adrenal cortical hypertrophy and basophilic adenomas of the pituitary gland.

Both prior to and after the description of Cushing, a considerable number of patients were considered under the category of "Achard-Thiers syndrome" or "the diabetes of bearded women".[5-8] In 1939, Shepardson and Shapiro presented a review of the 17 such cases from the literature.[9] Many of them were really suffering from Cushing's syndrome as we recognize it today. With the advance in our knowledge, the tendency among endocrinologists has been to ignore the so-called entity, "diabetes of the bearded woman", and to classify the patients with hirsutism and diabetes either as cases of Cushing's syndrome or as instances of simple coincidence of idiopathic hirsutism with diabetes mellitus. We believe the syndrome should be recognized as one of hyperandrogenism and diabetes and not as Cushing's disease.

Although decreased sensitivity to the hypoglycemic effects of insulin is the rule in obesity,[10,11] only obese people who are otherwise at 'high risk' appear to develop non-insulin-dependent diabetes mellitus.[12]

Clinical manifestations

The Archard-Thiers syndrome is a relatively rare condition. It has been described only in the female, usually over 30 years of age, and is characterized by the association of four major symptoms: obesity, diabetes, hirsutism and hypertension. No tendency to familial incidence has thus far been reported.

The obesity is usually prominent, being generalized. Fat accumulation occurs not only on the trunk, neck and face, but also involves the extremities.

The diabetes mellitus is of the relatively stable, moderately insulin-resistant type, commonly found in the overweight adult patient. Often, the diabetic stage is subclinical or latent, the classical symptoms being absent, and the diagnosis is made incidentally through laboratory procedures. There is no tendency to development of acidosis or diabetic coma. The complications are those of chronic, degenerative vascular changes associated with any type of diabetes that is present for a prolonged period of time.

The hirsutism is especially marked on the face, with moustache and beard that may require daily shaving. Excessive hair growth on the rest of the body is usually less intense or even absent. Other signs of virilization, like clitoral hypertrophy, receding hairline and deepening voice, may sometimes be found. The hypertension is moderate; the systolic pressure is more significantly increased than is the diastolic. Clinically, its behavior and complications resemble the benign type of essential hypertension. Menstrual disorders, although frequent, are not constant. Often the patients complain of oligomenorrhea or secondary amenorrhea, but a history of regular menses is occasionally obtained. The face, except for the obese appearance, shows no special characteristics. There is occasionally a plethoric facies. The skin may be oily with varying degree of acne. The pigment is eutrophic, without any evidence of deterioration due to increased protein catabolism. The only striae (stretch marks) to be found are of the white type resulting from excessive skin distension.

The major symptoms of this syndrome have their onset at different ages. A tendency to obesity may be noted from childhood or adolescence. Hirsutism frequently dates back to the epoch of the menarche and increases during the years that follow. The development of the diabetic stage or the onset of the elevated blood pressure are difficult to establish with accuracy since these

features are casually discovered by the physician.
The clinical evaluations of six patients are described in Table 1.

Laboratory procedures

The fasting blood sugar level may be elevated and glycosuria may be found. In any instance, a marked decrease in carbohydrate tolerance is evident when a glucose tolerance test is performed. The insulin tolerance test frequently reveals a diminished sensitivity to insulin. Serum electrolytes (Na^+, K^+, Cl^-, and HCO_3^-) are normal. Hematologic findings show no abnormal deviations directly related with the syndrome. Fasting eosinophil counts usually were found to be within normal limits. X-ray studies of the genito-urinary tract combined with presacral or peri-renal insufflations may suggest at times a certain degree of bilateral adrenal enlargement, but usually fail to reveal variations beyond normal limits in the size of the adrenal glands. Evidence of demineralization by X-ray study was lacking.

Discussion

Is the Achard-Thiers syndrome a distinctive clinical entity? A careful comparative analysis of Cushing's and Achard-Thiers syndromes reveals significant differences. In the Achard-Thiers syndrome there is an absence of symptoms resulting from the exaggerated anti-anabolic effect on protein metabolism, such as osteoporosis, muscle wasting, atrophic skin, purplish striae, weakness, hemorrhagic diathesis, protuberant abdomen (weak rectus muscles) and droopy upper lip (weak masseter muscles). In Achard-Thiers syndrome the face is not moon-shaped. Obesity is generalized, including the extremities; serum cortisol and testosterone are within normal limits; eosinophil count is rarely depressed and serum electrolytes are normal. Evidence against common etiologic factors for both Cushing and Achard-Thiers syndromes is therefore too strong to be ignored.

Frequently, cases of Achard-Thiers syndrome have been considered to be a mere coincidence of diabetes mellitus, idiopathic hirsutism and essential hypertension in obese patients. The expressions 'diathesis' or 'constitutional tendency' are employed to designate such associations of functional and metabolic disturbances but, in any case, they merely serve to expose our lack of knowledge. The excessive obesity characteristic of Achard-Thiers syndrome cannot be wholly regarded as only due to increased food intake, considering the relatively poor effect of low caloric diets upon the weight of these patients. Genetically determined hypersensitivity of the hair follicle apparatus could explain mild forms of hirsutism, but not the more advanced

Table 1 Clinical Data in 6 cases of Achard-Thiers Syndrome

Case No.	1 (A. E.)	2 (F. J.)*	3 (V. G.)	4 (D. A.)	5 (I. A.)	6 (J. S.)
AGE	36 yr.	36 yr.	56 yr.	26 yr.	32 yr.	30 yr.
RACE	W	W	W	W	W	W
OBESITY	Generalised	Generalised	Generalised	Generalised	Generalised	Generalised
HIRSUTISM	Moderate on face and body	Moderate on face and body	Heavy on face, none on body	Heavy on face and body	Heavy on face, slight on body	Heavy on face, moderate on body
AGE AT WHICH DIABETES WAS RECOGNIZED	35 yr.	35 yr.	56 yr.	26 yr.	26 yr.	29 yr.
BLOOD PRESSURE	155/100	180/120	170/80	165/95	130/80	175/110
MENSES	Oligomenorrhea	Normal	Regular menses until menopause at 44th year	Secondary amenorrhea	Regular menses until 32nd yr.	Oligomenorrhea
CLITORIS	Slightly enlarged	Normal	Normal	Slightly enlarged	Slightly enlarged	Slightly enlarged
STRIAE CUTANEA	White striae	White striae	White striae	No	No	No
PLETHORA	Yes	No	No	No	No	No
OTHER	Weakness	—	—	Father and mother were diabetic	Cholelithiasis	Retinitis pigmentosa

*–Symptoms 8 months after unilateral adrenalectomy.

signs of virilization. The mechanisms leading to the so-called 'essential hypertension' are polemic and subject to speculation.

Finally, it may be claimed that Achard-Thiers syndrome represents a mixed form of Cushing's syndrome and adrenogenital syndrome, in which the over-production of androgens compensates and diminishes the anti-anabolic effects of the glucocorticoids. Such mixed forms however, are usually associated with adrenal carcinoma and show considerably elevated serum levels of cortisol, testosterone and dehydroepiandrosterone (DHA).

It has been our purpose to call attention to this interesting symptomatic complex, the so-called 'diabetes of bearded women' or Achard-Thiers syndrome. It cannot at this point be finally determined whether or not such an entity exists, but in view of data and arguments now available, we feel that the syndrome may be clinically differentiated from other known endocrinopathies and therefore should be the subject of further consideration and clarification (Figs. 1 and 2).

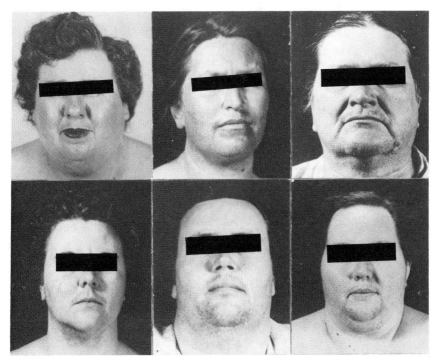

Figure 1. The facial appearance of six patients diagnosed as Achard-Thiers syndrome.

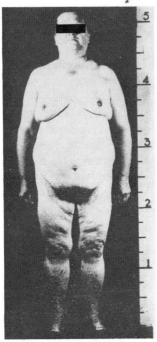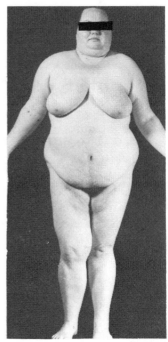

Figure 2. A and B. Two patients with Achard-Thiers syndrome. Note the generalized obesity and absence of purplish striae.

Differential diagnosis

Actually, the diagnosis of Achard-Thiers syndrome is made in the presence of generalized obesity, hirsutism, and diabetes mellitus, provided that the other recognizable diseases can be excluded as the causative factor in the symptomatology. Hypertension is also a very common finding.

A guide for differential diagnosis is presented in Table 2. Similarities and differences with Cushing's syndrome have already been discussed. The adrenogenital syndrome shows a much more advanced picture of virilization with high serum testosterone and lacks the obesity and diminished carbohydrate tolerance. In the congenital variety, hypertension is occasionally present, but the genital anomalies, the increased serum 17-hydroxyprogesterone, and the history of the disease should leave little confusion. Androgen producing tumors of the ovary are rare and should be ruled out. More difficult is the differentiation between Achard-Thiers syndrome and the Stein-Leventhal syndrome which presents the clinical association of obesity, hirsutism, and menstrual disorders in young or middle-aged women. Diabetes and hypertension would prove an acceptable diagnostic criteria for the former. The Stein-Leventhal syndrome is reviewed elsewhere in this book.

	Achard-Thiers Syndrome	Cushing's Syndrome	Stein-Leventhal Syndrome	Congenital Adrenogenital Syndrome in the Adult Female	Acquired Adrenogenital Syndrome in the Adult Female
STATURE	Normal	Normal	Normal	Short	Normal
OBESITY	Generalized	Limited to face and trunk	Generalized		
DIABETES	Present	Usually present			
HYPERTENSION	Frequent	Frequent			
HIRSUTISM	Mild	Mild	Mild to severe	Severe	Severe
MENSTRUAL DISORDERS	Usually oligomenorrhea	Usually oligomenorrhea	Usually functional amenorrhea	Primary amenorrhea	Secondary amenorrhea
EXTERNAL GENITALIA	Clitoris sometimes enlarged	Clitoris enlarged rarely	Clitoris enlarged rarely	Intersexual genitalia	Clitoris clearly enlarged
MUSCULAR SYSTEM	Normal	Atrophic	Normal	Hypertrophic	Hypertrophic
MOON FACE	Absent	Present	Absent	Absent	Absent
PLETHORA	Rare	Frequent	Absent	Absent	Absent
STRIAE CUTANEA	White type	Purplish type	White type	Absent	Absent
FRIABILITY OF CAPILLARIES	Normal	Increased	Normal	Normal	Normal
WEAKNESS	—	Yes	—	—	—
OSTEOPOROSIS	—	Yes	—	—	—
EDEMA	—	Occasionally	—	—	—
PSYCHIC SYMPTOMS	—	Frequent	—	—	—
EOSINOPHIL COUNT	Usually normal	Usually less than 100/cu. mm.	Normal	Normal	Normal

Summary

Attention is drawn to an interesting symptom-complex, the Achard-Thiers syndrome. The diagnosis should be made by exclusion, especially after Cushing's disease has been eliminated. It cannot at this point be finally determined whether such an entity exists, nor what abnormality in steroid secretion and/or metabolism is present. It may well be that the syndrome is merely the result of coincidental diabetes mellitus and hirsutism.

ACANTHOSIS NIGRICANS

Acanthosis nigricans is a relatively rare disease: a hyperpigmented verrucous, velvety lesion involving the flexural creases in the axilla, groin, antecubital and popliteal fossae and the nape of the neck. Obesity, hypertrichosis and diabetes are frequent manifestations. Polycystic ovarian disease or other endocrine disorders may be present. The physician often is hard-put to rule out Cushing's disease, but the thick skin, the generalized obesity, and no evidence of muscle wasting immediately stamps this entity as not Cushing's disease. A typical case history follows:

A 15-year-old girl was hospitalized for evaluation of hirsutism, amenorrhea and obesity. Menses began at 13 years of age, but had always been irregular, lasting five days with intervals of seven to nine months between periods. Her last menstrual period occurred nine months before admission. The patient denied use of oral contraceptives. Facial hair and acne had increased in the past one and a half years. She had always been large, but her weight had increased dramatically during the preceding three years. There was also a recent history of extreme thirst and excessive urination. For a number of years, she had noted thickened, dark skin on the back of her neck, and in the axilla and groin.

Findings on the physical examination: weight, 216 lbs; height, 65 inches; blood pressure, 180/110 mm Hg. There was severe acne on the face and back, facial hirsutism (Fig. 3a) and excessive body hair, acanthosis nigricans of the back of the neck, axilla and groin, and a massively enlarged abdomen with purple striae (Fig. 3b). The skin was not thin and there was no evidence of protein wasting. Pelvic examination revealed an enlarged clitoris (1.5 cm), male escutcheon, nulliparous cervix and no adnexal masses. Fern test of the cervical mucus showed no estrogen effect; maturation index revealed 81% parabasal cells, 19% intermediate cells, and no superficial cells, which indicates low estrogen effect.

X-rays of the skull, sella turcica, chest and abdomen were normal. Ultrasound revealed a retroverted uterus which measured 6 cm from the cervix to the fundus; the ovaries could not be definitely visualized. Intravenous pyelogram (IVP) was normal.

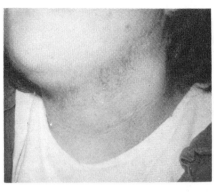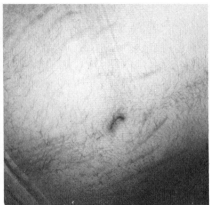

Figure 3. A. Pseudo-Cushing's syndrome in a 15-year-old girl with hypertension, diabetes mellitus, marked obesity and elevated cortisol, free testosterone and testosterone levels (LH:FSH ratio elevated). Note the degree of hirsutism.
B. Photograph of the patient's abdomen, demonstrating striae and hirsutism.

Laboratory blood studies revealed polycythemia (increased red blood cells), eosinopenia (abnormally small number of eosinophil cells), lymphopenia (reduction in lymphocytes), diabetes (elevated glucose levels). Endocrine function tests revealed elevated urinary 17-ketosteroids, plasma testosterone, free testosterone, serum LH, and FSH levels. The plasma cortisol levels were elevated (31 μg per dl. at 8 a.m., 29 μg dl. at 4 p.m.). After the patient received 1 mg of dexamethasone at midnight, plasma cortisol at 8 a.m. was 22 μg per ml. Plasma ACTH at 8 a.m. was 35.3 pg ml (normal: 20 to 100 pg per ml).

Because of the elevated cortisol levels, polycythemia, lymphopenia, eosinopenia, diabetes, hypertension and hirsutism, a more complete dexamethasone suppression test was indicated. Accordingly, on days 1 and 2, 24-hour urine collections for 17-hydroxysteroids and 17-ketosteroids were obtained. Then on days 3 and 4, the patient was given 0.5 mg of dexamethasone every six hours for eight doses; on days 5 and 6, she received 2 mg of dexamethasone every six hours for eight doses (Table 2). Plasma cortisol levels were obtained at 8 a.m. on days 3, 4, and 6.

Even though the fasting plasma cortisol values were in the range that suggested Cushing's disease, the patient's appearance (generalized obesity, thick skin and lack of signs of muscle wasting or weakness) was considered more diagnostically significant than the cortisol levels. Before further investigation, it was decided to observe the patient and begin treatment for probable Stein-Leventhal syndrome (high LH:FSH ratio).

Table 3 Dexamethasone Suppression Test in Illustrative Case

Day	Plasma cortisol at 8 a.m.	Urinary 17-hydroxysteroids		Urinary 17-ketosteroids		Creatinine (mg. per dl.)	Total volume (ml.)
		mg. per 24 hours	mg. per Gm. of creatinine	mg. per 24 hours	mg. per Gm. of creatinine		
1	20µg. per dl.	9.3	4.7	15.2	7.6	2.0	615
2		6.1	5.1	12.6	10.5	1.2	390
*3							
**4	12µg. per dl.	3.4	2.3	10.6	7.1	1.5	450
**5	1.3µg. per dl. (note suppression)	2.8	3.5	5.1	6.4	0.8	305
**6		8.5	2.1	16.6	4.2	4.0	1,400
7	1.0µg. per dl.						

Urinary 17-hydroxysteroids were suppressed after two days of dexamethasone administration. Urinary 17-hydroxysteroids and 17-ketosteroids appeared to increase on day 6; however, this was due to an increase in urinary creatinine and volume. When expressed as mg. per Gm. of creatinine, they remained suppressed. This demonstrates the importance of the urinary creatinine determination when interpreting urinary steroid excretion. (In Cushing's syndrome, urinary 17-hydroxysteroids are usually more than 7 mg. per Gm. of creatinine and do not suppress to less than 2.5 mg. per Gm. of creatinine after dexamethasone.)

*—Dexamethasone, 0.5 mg. every six hours on days 3 and 4.
**—Dexamethasone, 2.0 mg. every six hours on days 5 and 6.

An oral contraceptive (Enovid-E) was prescribed for 21 days each month, along with a weight-reducing regimen (1,000-calorie low carbohydrate diet). Six months later, the patient had lost 42 pounds, blood glucose levels had returned to normal, blood pressure was greatly reduced (142/90), and serum testosterone and free testosterone levels were normal[12].

Although features of this case were strongly suggestive of Cushing's syndrome, the diagnosis was evidently "not Cushing's disease" but one of acanthosis nigricans.

References

1. Achard, M. C. and Thiers, M. J. Le virilisme pilaire et son association à l'insuffisance glycolytique (Diabète des femmes à barbe). Bull Acad de Med Par 86:51, 1927

2. Kraus: Deutsch med Wchnschr 39:298, 1913

3. Tuffier, M. Bull Acad de med Par 71:726, 1914

4. Cushing, H. The basophil adenomas of the pituitary body and their clinical manifestation (Pituitary basophilism). Bull Johsns Hopkins Hosp 50:137, 1932

5. Brown, W. H. A case of pluriglandular syndrome: "Diabetes of bearded women". Lancet 2:1022, 1928

6. Weil, M. P., Weissman-Netter, R. and Renaudeaux, M. Hirsutisme et diabète. À l'occasion d'une observation personnelle. Gaz med de France 15:373, 1930

7. Shallow, T. A. Adrenal tumor producing the Achard-Thiers' syndrome. Ann Surg 98:297, 1933

8. Duncan, G. G. and Fetter, F. Suprarenal tumor-hirsutism-diabetes. Med Clin North America 18:261, 1934

9. Shepardson, H. C. and Shapiro, E. The diabetes of bearded women (Suprarenal tumor, diabetes and hirsutism). A clinical correlation of the function of the suprarenal cortex in carbohydrate metabolism. Endocrinol 24:237, 1939

10. Wilder, R. M., Kernohaw, J. W. and Perker, H. L. et al: Symposium: polyglandular dyscrasias involving abnormalities of sexual characteristics. Proc Staff Meet Mayo Clinic 8:97, 1933

11. Bush, I. E. and Mahesh, V. B. Adrenal hyperfunction with sudden onset of hirsutism. J Endocrinol 18:1, 1959

12. Rincon, J., Greenblatt, R. B. and Schwartz, R. P., Not Cushing's syndrome. Am Fam Phys 5 (May):77, 1979

7
The Ovary as a Source of Androgens
A. The Polycystic Ovary
B. Masculinizing Ovarian Tumors

Robert B. Greenblatt, M.D.
R. Don Gambrell, JR., M.D.

The mystique surrounding the polycystic ovary has beguiled gynecologists and endocrinologists for many years. When Galen (2nd century) designated the ovary as the female testicle, he presciently served notice that the female gonad was not unlike a testis. The large pale ovary, a descriptive term employed by Albright for the polycystic ovary of Stein-Leventhal, indeed bears a resemblance to the testicle. Such ovaries have the capacity to produce abnormal amounts of androgens, so that the sobriquet "the androgenic ovary" is not inappropriate. The typical woman with this syndrome usually presents with a normal age of menarche, coincident with the onset of unwanted hair growth, usually followed by menstrual irregularity ranging from absence to excessive menstruation.

The polycystic ovary was first alluded to by Chereau in 1844 when he described sclerocystic ovaries. A host of conditions was attributed to them, and later in the century removal of the ovaries became a widely used therapeutic procedure. In 1896, Waldo applied the principle of partial resection rather than removal, and several years later, Findley, in discussing cystic degeneration of the ovary, felt that wedge-resection was of great value.[1,2] Nonetheless, he did not hesitate to remove both ovaries. In 1910, Forgue and Massabuau reviewed the subject of sclerocystic ovaries and suggested that an appropriate designation would be "microcystic ovaries".[3] They concluded that the precise anatomic lesions of the microcystic ovary are poorly understood. In 1935, Stein and Leventhal reported on a series of cases with absence of menses and bilaterally enlarged polycystic ovaries.[4] The correlation of the symptomatology, means of diagnosis, and wedge-resection as the ideal mode of therapy which bears their names.

HISTOPATHOLOGY

Is there a specific pathology for the polycystic ovary? In general, the gross appearance of the polycystic ovary is not specific, for a similar picture may be seen in other conditions associated with anovulation, such as Cushing's syndrome, congenital adrenal hyperplasia, hypothyroidism, acromegaly, and hyperprolactinemia.

The gross appearance of the polycystic ovary is quite characteristic. It is usually elongated, one and a half to two times normal, with a smooth pearly-white surface or tunica (Fig. 1). On sectioning, numerous pea-sized cysts, filled with clear fluid, occupy the thickened cortex (Fig. 2). In some instances the ovary is not enlarged, i.e., the small microcystic ovary. The cortex is often fibrotic and has been mislabeled as a thickened ovarian capsule, and the question has often been asked, "Is the thick sclerotic 'capsule' a deterrent to the ovulatory process?"

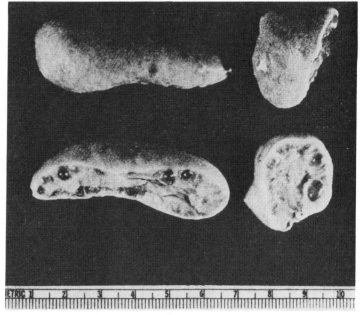

Figure 1.   Wedge section of typically elongated polycystic ovaries. Note the subcortical microcysts and the well-defined tunica albuginea.

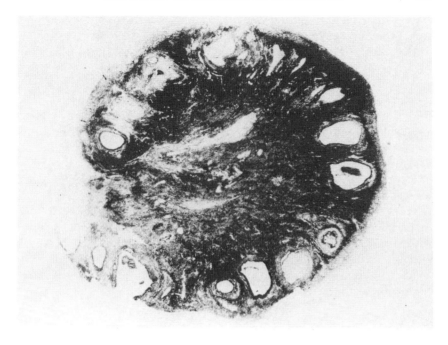

Figure 2. Low-power view of histologic section from a polycystic ovary illustrative of the multiple microcysts, the thickened cortex, the dense medullary stroma.

The myth that the thick sclerotic tunica acts as a mechanical barrier to ovulation is perpetuated in many textbooks. The distinguished Viennese gynecologist, the late Prof. Antoine, as recently as 1971 wrote that among the causes of infertility "there may be anatomical reasons like in the Stein-Leventhal syndrome with its thickened tunica albuginea."[5] For this reason, operations for stripping the capsule or techniques for ovarian eversion were devised. Some believe that ovulation takes place after wedge-resection along the weakened approximated edges of the ovary. Greenblatt performed unilateral oophorectomy (removal of one ovary) in five patients with the classical syndrome, resulting in cyclic ovulations from the contralateral ovary in four patients despite the so-called thickened capsule.[6] Because clomiphene, human gonadotropins, and glucocorticoids may readily induce ovulation, the thick 'capsule' may no longer be considered a deterrent to ovulation.

HYPOTHALAMIC-PITUITARY AXIS AND THE POLYCYSTIC OVARY

Is the polycystic ovary primarily a hypothalamic-pituitary disorder? Before this question can be answered, the following observations need to be taken into account.

1.   Women with this syndrome occasionally ovulate under stress conditions. This was strikingly brought to the fore when in 1958 a 32-year-old
woman with classical Stein-Leventhal syndrome was hospitalized for
wedge-resection in the hope of resolving her infertility problem. At the time
of admission, she had not menstruated in nine months. Laparotomy revealed
typically elongated ovaries with a thick pearl-like 'capsule' and a small fresh
corpus luteum bulging the lateral extremity of the left ovary. Wedge-
resection was performed on each ovary. The histopathology was in conso-
nance with that usually found, except for the fresh corpus luteum and an old
hyalinized corpus albicans in one of the sections from the right ovary.
Incidentally, the patient had regular ovulatory menses for 16 years following
surgery.[6]

Support for spontaneous ovulations in stress situations was obtained in our
study of 30 women with infrequent or absent menses who were hospitalized
with Stein-Leventhal syndrome. Five ovulated before clomiphene therapy or
wedge-resection could be undertaken. Figure 3 is illustrative of one such case;
on the morning of admission, both FSH and LH values were at levels
compatible with the ovulatory surge.[7]

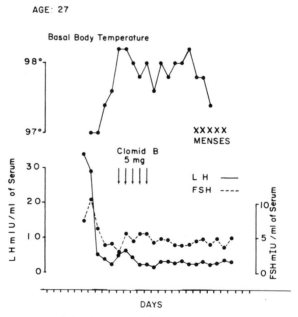

Figure 3.   Spontaneous ovulation in a 27-year-old nulligravida on admission to hospital. Note
elevated LH and FSH values and typical rise in basal body temperature. Eventual wedge-
resection revealed enlarged polycystic ovaries histologically compatible with Stein-Leventhal
syndrome. (Reproduced with permission from Gambrell, R. D., et al: Obstet Gynecol 38:857,
1971)

2. Polycystic ovaries frequently contain large quantities of androgens.[10] These androgens may have a direct inhibitory effect on ovarian follicular development and may also alter gonadotropin secretion by their effect along with that of the peripherally produced estrogens on the hypothalamic-pituitary system. Wedge-resection effectively reduces ovarian androgens and their peripheral conversion products and results in the restoration of cyclic ovulation. This would be difficult to explain if a hypothalamic-pituitary defect were present.

3. Typical polycystic ovaries may be found in the presence of a virilizing adrenal adenoma, and in the contralateral ovary in women harboring an ovarian androgen-producing tumor.

One may conclude from the above observations that the pituitary-ovarian axis remains more or less intact in the polycystic ovary. Endogenous androgens in certain virilizing syndromes have a direct or indirect effect on the ovary. Excess androgens or perhaps their ready conversion to estrogens appear to affect the higher brain centers of the hypothalamus. Chronic anovulation is a characteristic of the polycystic ovary.

The pituitary gland of women with polycystic ovaries may have heightened sensitivity to hypothalamic luteinizing releasing hormone (gnRH) to account for the exaggerated pulsatile release of LH. The enhanced sensitivity may be due to the high levels of estrogens circulating in these patients because estrogens are known to increase the sensitivity of the pituitary gland in experimental animals. This results in an elevated LH:FSH ratio, hence the term 'hyperluteinizing syndrome' has crept into the literature. Yen believes that only these women with inappropriate LH secretion can truly be said to have Stein-Leventhal syndrome.[8] On the other hand, we have encountered several women with classical Stein-Leventhal syndrome who had very low circulating estrogens, as evidenced by castrate vaginal smears. Furthermore, Gambrell et al feel that there are many instances of the polycystic ovary syndrome in which the LF:FSH ratio is not disturbed.[7] Other investigators feel as we do, that there are two types of polycystic ovaries: one with a high, the other with a normal LH:FSH ratio. In fact, a third type has come into the picture and that is the so-called pseudopolycystic ovary with prolactinemia (Table 1).

POLYCYSTIC OVARY AS A SOURCE OF EXCESSIVE ANDROGENS

Early reports of elevated urinary 17-ketosteroids in the polycystic ovary syndrome invariably implicated the adrenal as the main source of excessive androgens. The possibility of the secretion of excessive androgens by the polycystic ovary was considered by Greenblatt as early as 1953,[9] by the demonstration of a decrease in 17-ketosteroids on wedge-resection or follow-

Table 1. Hormone Serum Assays in Eight Patients with Stein-Leventhal Syndrome and Presumed Adenoma of the Pituitary Gland

	Group A (SLS with Hyperprolactinemia)				Group B (SLS without Hyperprolactinemia)			
	J.M.‡ 24 yrs	K.A.‡ 24 yrs	R.S. 29 yrs	G.I. 18 yrs	A.D. 18 yrs	O.G. 27 yrs	G.B. 27 yrs	W.T. 29 yrs
PRL, ng/ml	55.7	51.2	45.7	7.4	20.3	6.9	22.5	16.4
FSH, mIU/ml	4.2	2.4	4.6	9.2	4.0	3.4	3.3	4.6
LH, mIU/ml	29.4	27.2	28.5	45.5	27.3	22.4	46.7	38.4
T, ng/ml	0.8	0.7	0.6	4.3	0.7	0.8	2.3	0.8
∇^4-A, ng/ml	0.9	2.8	0.7	1.9	2.8	3.6	2.6	1.3
DHA, µg/ml	1.3	1.4	1.4	2.2	2.1	1.5	2.7	1.1
E_2, pg/ml	20.5	25.8	36.4	18.5	52.9	44.4	43.1	53.5

‡ Galactorrhea

(Reproduced with permission from Greenblatt, R. B. Inappropriate lactation in men and women – the role of prolactin secretion, in Bravo, A. A. (ed) : A Temas Actuales de Ginecologia Obstetricia. Mexico, 1979)

ing removal of the ovaries. Similar findings were made in later years by other investigators. However, wedge-resection failed to induce ovulatory menses in occasional cases despite a lowering of urinary 17-ketosteroids, yet ovulation could be induced by the administration of glucocorticoids in some of these patients. The adrenal component could not be overlooked.

Patients with polycystic ovary syndrome complex with excessive androgens could represent an adrenal or an ovarian disorder, or one involving both. Thus, corticosteroid therapy might induce ovulatory menses, while wedge-resection could do likewise in the same patient (Fig. 4). The cause of the high levels of androgens in women with polycystic ovary syndrome is not clear. The activity of the adrenal glands can be suppressed by the use of corticosteroids, yet the elevated levels of testosterone and ∇^4/androstenedione persist, reflecting ovarian production of the steroids. Direct sampling of adrenal and ovarian vein blood has shown that the ovarian effluent has the highest concentration of testosterone and androstenedione while levels of dehydroepiandrosterone are much higher in adrenal vein blood than in peripheral blood.

CONFIRMATION OF EXCESSIVE SECRETION OF ANDROGENS BY POLYCYSTIC OVARIES IN OTHER STUDIES

In the 1960s, the secretion of excessive androgens by the polycystic ovary was a new concept and therefore adequate confirmation was needed. This was done in the study of steroid content of ovarian tissue and ovarian venous blood. The normal ovary contained only small quantities of ∇^4androstenedione. The ovaries of patients with the polycystic ovary syndrome contained large quantities of either ∇^4androstenedione and 17α-hydroxyprogesterone and/or dehydroepiandrosterone. The secretion of large quantities of ∇^4androstenedione and dehydroepiandrosterone by the polycystic ovary was amply confirmed by the isolation of large quantities of these compounds from ovarian venous blood.

MEASUREMENT OF BLOOD ANDROGENS

The measurement of various androgens in the blood of hirsute patients with the polycystic ovary syndrome was carried out by several investigators with emphasis on testosterone measurements. Although in a large number of cases blood testosterone was elevated, it was nevertheless found to be within normal limits in a substantial number of hirsute patients. Hirsute patients were found to have significant elevations not only in testosterone, but also dehydroepiandrosterone, ∇^4-androstenedione, 5α-dihydrotestosterone, and 17α-hydroxyprogesterone (Fig. 5). The elevation in these steroids is in

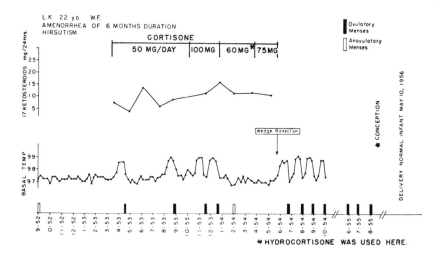

Figure 4. Patient, L. K. Note sporadic ovulations on cortisone and the establishment of regular ovulatory menses following wedge-resection.
(Reproduced with permission from Greenblatt, R. B. *The Hirsute Female.* Springfield, IL., Charles C. Thomas, 1963, p 158)

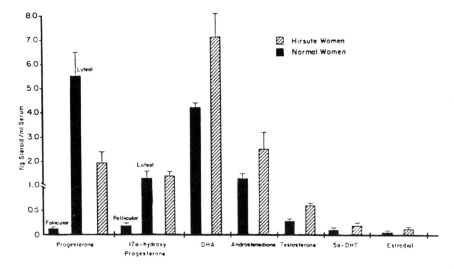

Figure 5. Peripheral blood steroids in 10 normal women and 13 hirsute women. Note elevation of dehydroepiandrosterone ∇^4androstenedione, and testosterone in hirsute women, 17α-hydroxyprogesterone and progesterone levels in hirsute women were comparable to those found in the luteal phase of normal women.
(Reproduced with permission from Greenblatt, R. B. and Mahesh, V. B. The androgenic polycystic ovary. In, *Hirsutism and Virilism: Pathogenesis, diagnosis, and management.* Greenblatt, R. B. and Mahesh, V. B. (eds). Boston, Wright, P. S. G., 1983, p 213)

agreement with the variety of steroids isolated from ovarian tissue and ovarian venous blood. Studies of peripheral blood steroids and urinary steroids have yielded valuable information regarding excessive androgen secretion in the polycystic ovary syndrome. However, whether the source of these androgens was the adrenal or the ovary has often been difficult to ascertain.

ETIOLOGIC FACTORS

The causes of the syndrome are still obscure. We have long maintained that the syndrome is triggered by an unusual adrenarche. Others also feel that it may arise as an adrenal disorder during the early phase of sexual maturation, resulting in a progressive increase of the secretion of androgens by this gland. The distorted androgen levels could then result in increased extraglandular conversion so that the resulting high levels of estrogen interfere with the release of gonadotropins and cause the imbalance typical of these patients. Hereditary factors may be involved in this syndrome.

MANAGEMENT

The goal of therapy in the woman with androgenic (microcystic) ovaries is either to decrease androgen production by the ovaries and/or adrenals in the hope of gradually lessening hirsutism or to induce ovulation in an attempt to overcome infertility.

Estrogens and oral contraceptives have been employed with a modicum of success in putting the ovary to rest and by increasing protein-binding sex globulin. By such a process it has been alleged that less free testosterone is available to stimulate the receptors of the pilosebaceous unit. Corticosteroids have also been used to suppress adrenal androgens, and corticoids may also dampen androgen production rates in idiopathic hirsutism and polycystic ovaries. The effectiveness of estrogens and corticoids in suppressing ovarian and adrenal androgens was amply shown in ovarian and adrenal vein catheterization studies as shown in Figure 6.

Allusion was previously made to psychogenic factors and also to the fact that corticosteroids may be employed to induce ovulation. When an analog of chlorotrianisene (Tace), known as MER-25, was made available for clinical trial, Tyler et al reported in 1960 that this antiestrogen successfully induced ovulation,[10] an observation later confirmed by others. This drug was removed from clinical investigation because of toxic reactions. About this time, another analog, MRL-41, also an antiestrogen, was made available for clinical trial as a possible oral contraceptive. It failed as such but proved eminently satisfactory as an ovulatory inducing agent. In 1961, Greenblatt et

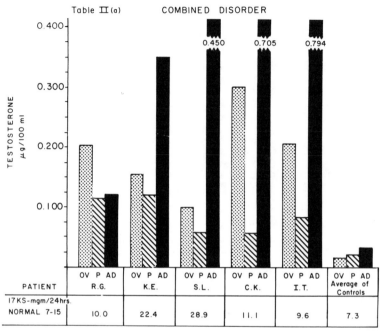

Figure 6.   Plasma testosterone values in three of eight hirsute patients with polycystic ovaries. In each patient, ovarian and adrenal vein testosterone obtained through femoral catheterization were higher than peripheral venous levels. In patient L.Mc. estrogen therapy resulted in ovarian and peripheral testosterone decrease to within normal limits while adrenal testosterone remained markedly elevated.

(Reproduced from Stahl, N. L., Teeslink, C. R. and Greenblatt, R. B. Ovarian, adrenal and peripheral testosterone levels in polycystic ovary syndrome. Am J Obstet Gynecol 117:194, 1973)

al reported that 28 or 36 amenorrheic women ovulated following a course of this agent, later known as clomiphene.[11] Clomiphene was employed in a variety of anovulatory conditions, and the best results were obtained in the treatment of Stein-Leventhal syndrome (Table 2).[12] Even women who responded with ovulatory menses to wedge-resection for only a few months, frequently were made to ovulate with clomiphene (Fig. 7). When clomiphene alone does not seem to work, then a few days later an intramuscular injection of 5,000 to 10,000 units of human chorionic gonadotrophin (hCG) may be administered. Clomiphene-resistant patients frequently respond to such a regimen.

As a last resort, one may use the readily available human menopausal gonadotropin, Pergonal, as employed by Lunenfeld et al (Fig. 8).[13] A warning should be sounded in the treatment of women with the polycystic ovary syndrome with either clomiphene or gonadotropins. The ovaries of such patients are quite sensitive and minimal dosages should be used to avoid the 'hyperstimulation syndrome'.

Table 2. Incidence of Presumably Ovulatory Cycles following Clomiphene*

	No. Patients	No. Cycles	Ovulation	Percentage
Patients treated	257	1331	962	72.7
Oligomenorrhea	87	418	343	82.0
Secondary amenorrhea	75	465	297	63.9
Primary amenorrhea	18	109	26	23.8
Stein-Leventhal	42	165	149	90.0
Dysfunctional uterine bleeding	35	174	147	84.5

* Dosages varied from 50 mg to 200 mg × 5 days. Occasionally up to 100 mg was given for 10 days.
(Modified from Greenblatt, R. B., et al: Excerpta Med Int Congr Ser 1964; 101:59)

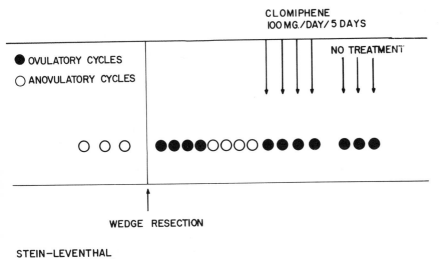

Figure 7. Following wedge-resection of the ovaries in a patient with Stein-Leventhal syndrome, four ovulatory menses occurred. Anovulatory menstrual periods again set in and Clomid therapy once again induced ovulatory menses; the patient continued to have ovulatory cycles after discontinuation of therapy.
(IBID)

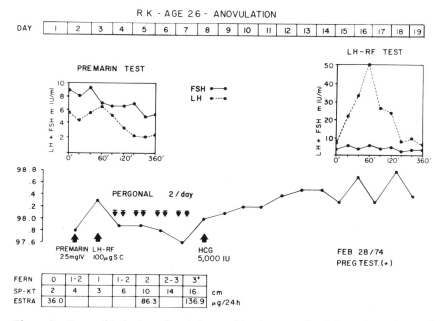

Figure 8. Pergonal induction of ovulation resulting in conception. Note prior to Pergonal therapy, a lowering of FSH and LH levels was obtained following 25 mg of intravenous Premarin and marked LH rise following 100 μg of LRF subcutaneously. Also note monitoring of Pergonal administration by fern formation and spinnbarkeit of cervical mucus, and urinary estrogen levels.
(IBID)

CONCLUSION

What assumptions may be drawn from the evidence at hand as to the pathogenesis of the polycystic ovary? We believe it is fair to say that the higher centers of the brain are influenced at the time of adrenarche by elevated circulating estrogens (peripherally converted from androgens) leading to a discordance in the hypothalamic-pituitary-ovarian axis. With the onset of the menarche, early signs of hairiness begin to appear, and irregular menstrual periods ensue. But, the very fact that under certain stress situations ovulation can take place is proof enough that the disturbance in the axis is functional and not organic.

Hirsute females are more responsive to a test dose of ACTH than normal women by secreting larger amounts of urinary 17-ketosteroids.[14] This feature may well be genetic since we have seen polycystic ovaries and marked hirsutism in several siblings. Study of blood obtained by catheterization of ovarian and adrenal veins revealed markedly elevated levels of androgens and particularly testosterone in women with polycystic ovaries in comparison with normal controls. Because of an inherent capacity of the adrenals, and perhaps the ovaries too, to produce excess androgens, it may be assumed that a chain of reactions is initiated which ultimately leads to the development of polycystic ovaries.

It appears then that an inherent capacity for androgen production by the adrenal upsets hypothalamic-pituitary-ovarian relationships. As a result, a steady state of discordant gonadotropin secretion stimulates the growth of a myriad of follicles, luteinizing the theca and often certain cellular elements in the stroma. As a consequence, the ovary usually enlarges and elongates; absence of ovulations is reflected in the smooth glistening 'capsule'. Priming the pituitary pump causes a derangement in orderly ovarian steroidogenesis, resulting in increased androgen production. Thus, the bourgeoning poly- or microcystic ovary becomes an 'androgenic ovary'.

MASCULINIZING OVARIAN TUMORS

The contribution of the ovaries in the production of androgens has been discussed. Ovarian tumors which produce excessive amounts of the so-called male hormones – the androgens – are rare, perhaps responsible for less than 0.1% of the cases of hirsutism and virilism. From the 3,500 ovarian tumors diagnosed at Johns Hopkins Medical School during the past 40 years, only 33 were classified as masculinizing ovarian tumors, or less than 1% of all ovarian tumors, which in themselves are unusual, if not rare.[15]. The onset of hirsutism, when caused by a tumor, differs from that caused by dysfunctional ovaries, such as the polycystic ovary of Stein-Leventhal. In the latter, development of hirsutism is gradual from adolescence onwards; in tumors, there is a rapid onset that may take place at any time in a woman's life.

Ovarian tumors have been classified as hormone producing and non-hormone producing. The hormones produced may either be estrogens or androgens, such as testosterone and androstenedione, or in rare cases, both estrogens and androgens. A few years ago, it was popular to classify these tumors according to the basic cell type; ovarian cells principally produced estrogens, such as granulosa or theca cells, or androgens, such as stroma cells, which resulted in classifying these tumors as non-virilizing or virilizing (masculinizing). It should be recalled that the cells lining the egg follicles are theca and granulosa cells, while cells in between the follicles are called stromal cells. The granulosa and theca cells primarily produce estrogens in the normal ovary, while the stromal cells produce mostly androgens, some of which are converted into estrogens. Thus, ovarian tumors were named according to the predominant cell type, such as *thecoma* for tumors composed of theca cells, and *granulosa cell tumors* when that type was predominant. Stromal cells may form tumors called arrhenoblastoma that have cells very similar to those in the male gonad, the testis.[16] This should not be surprising since in early embryonic development, the gonad is neither female (ovary) nor male (testicle) but changes into ovaries or testes at about the third month of fetal life.

With more accurate methods of measuring hormones, it has been realized in recent years that the basic cell type of the ovarian tumor may produce either estrogens or androgens, even both hormones. Therefore, whether an ovarian tumor is non-masculinizing or masculinizing depends more on the clinical features rather than the appearance under the microscope. Instances have even been reported where cancer spreading from other parts of the body, such as the intestinal tract, has induced increased androgen production. The presence of a benign cyst, called the dermoid cyst which arises from germ cells (the egg), and which may or may not per se produce androgenic hormones, is usually associated with a polycystic ovary on the other (contralateral) side. This ovary may become an androgenic ovary and be the source of the agent producing unwanted hair.

Tumors of the ovary may be benign or of low risk for malignancy; others are highly malignant. It is important to remove these masculinizing tumors as soon as a diagnosis is made. The clinical features are very similar to the virilizing adrenal tumors, except an ovarian enlargement can usually be felt on examination. Some masculinizing ovarian tumors are quite small, specifically those arising from the hilus cells. Usually, the patients with tumors are not just hirsute, but have other masculine characteristics as well, such as enlargement of the clitoris, increased muscle mass leading to a masculine body type, and cephalic alopecia (male-pattern baldness). Blood testosterone levels are frequently markedly increased along with other androgens, such as androstenedione. Androgen metabolites in the urine, the 17-ketosteroids, are also increased considerably. This is in contrast with the polycystic ovary syndrome where blood testosterone is usually normal or only slightly elevated, while urinary 17-ketosteroids are almost always normal in patients with the Stein-Leventhal syndrome.

Other important clinical distinctions between polycystic ovaries and masculinizing ovarian tumors include age of onset. Hirsutism secondary to polycystic ovaries usually has its onset at or soon after adolescence where virilizing tumors have a more rapid onset in later life. With both tumors and polycystic ovaries, menstrual periods may cease, and rarely recur until the tumor is surgically removed. Voice changes may also occur with masculinizing ovarian tumors, similar to what a male goes through at puberty, with crackling first followed by a deepening, more male-like voice. Specialized tests such as ultrasound of the pelvis may detect a unilateral ovarian enlargement, where polycystic ovaries are usually symetrically enlarged. Laparoscopy, or actually looking at the ovaries with a telescope-like instrument inserted through the abdominal wall under anesthesia, can usually differentiate tumors from polycystic ovaries.

As stated previously, treatment is surgical removal of the tumor since no medications are available which would suppress androgen production by an ovarian tumor. Although many masculinizing ovarian tumors are benign, some are malignant. Since this cannot be determined without microscopic examination of the tumor, they should all be excised. The opposite ovary should be examined internally at surgery by incising it and looking for other small tumors because on occasion both ovaries may be involved. Once the source of excessive androgens is removed, menstrual periods usually resume, and some of the hirsutism may resolve; however, the masculinization may persist for many years, if not indefinitely.

References

1. Waldo, Quoted by Schockaert, J. A. Considerations au sujet sept cas de syndrome de Stein-Leventhal-Cohen. C. R Soc Fr Gynecol 25:402, 1955
2. Findley, P. Cystic degeneration of the ovary. Am J Obstet Dis Women Child 49:762, 1904
3. Forgue, E. and Massabuau G. Les lesions et la pathogenie de la degenerescense microkystique des ovaries. Press Med 18:412, 1910
4. Stein, I. F. and Leventhal, M. L. Amenorrhea associated with bilateral polycystic ovaries. Am J Obstet Gynecol 29:181, 1935
5. Antoine, T. Etiology of female fertility disturbances in normal and pathologic human ovaries. Obstet Gynecol 24:667, 1964
6. Greenblatt, R. B. The polycystic ovary syndrome. Md State Med J 10:120, 1961
7. Gambrell, R. D., Greenblatt, R. B. and Mahesh, V. B. Serum gonadotropins and ancillary studies in Stein-Leventhal syndrome treated with clomiphene citrate. Obstet Gynecol 38:850, 1971
8. Yen S. C. C., Vela, P. and Rankin, J. Inappropriate secretion of FSH and LH in polycystic ovarian disease. J Clin Endocrinol Metab 30:435, 1970
9. Greenblatt, R. B. Cortisone in treatment of the hirsute woman. Am J Obstet Gynecol 66:700, 1953
10. Tyler, E. T., Olson, H. J. and Gotlib, M. H. The induction of ovulation with antiestrogen. Int J Fertil 5:429, 1961
11. Greenblatt, R. B., Barfield, W. E. and Jungck, E. C. et al: Induction of ovulation with MRL-41. JAMA 12:121, 1961
12. Greenblatt, R. B., Zarate, A. and Mahesh, V. B. La induccion de la ovulation en el humano con citrato de clomifen. Excerpta Medica Int Congr Ser 101:59, 1964
13. Lunenfeld, B., Menzi, A. and Volet, B. Clinical effect of human postmenopausal gonadotropins. In, Fuchs First International Congress of Endocrinology, 1960, p 295
14. Lloyd, C. W. Studies of adrenal function of hirsute women. In, The Hirsute Female, Greenblatt, R. B. (ed). Springfield, IL., Charles C. Thomas, 1963, p 88
15. Woodruff, J. D. and Parmley, T. H. Virilizing ovarian tumors. In, Hirsutism and Virilism, Mahesh, V. B. and Greenblatt, R. B. (eds). Boston, John Wright PSG Inc, 1983, pp 129-158
16. Greenblatt, R. B., Mahesh, V. B. and Gambrell, R. D. Jr. Arrenoblastoma: Three case reports. Obstet Gynecol 39:567, 1972

8
The Adrenal as a Source of Androgens

Anthony E. Karpas, M.D.

The adrenal glands are situated just above each kidney and are about the size of a walnut. Each adrenal consists of an inner portion (medulla) and an outer portion (cortex). The medulla is connected to the sympathetic nervous system and produces adrenalin (epinephrine) and noradrenalin (norepinephrine) in response to stress. The cortex produces three main sets of hormones: glucocorticoids, mineralocorticoids and androgens. Production of these hormones also occurs in response to stress situations, thus the adrenal may rightly be called the stress glands of the body.

The relationships between androgens and hirsutism has been elegantly outlined elsewhere in this book. Since our discussion is limited to the effect of the adrenal glands on hair growth, we will concentrate only on the adrenal cortex which is a significant contributor of androgens in the female.[1-7]

THE ADRENAL CORTEX

The three main groups of hormones produced by the adrenal cortex are similar in structure, and are known as steroid hormones: (1) glucocorticoids (cortisol) play an important role in glucose and lipid metabolism; (2) mineralocorticoids (aldosterone) are involved in the balance of water, sodium, and potassium in the blood, as well as for blood pressure regulation; (3) androgens are anabolic steroid hormones responsible for muscle build-up and sexual function.

The most important hormone secreted by the adrenal, in terms of the body's inability to function without it, is cortisol. Cortisol levels are monitored by the brain in much the same way as a thermostat works. The brain controls cortisol production by stimulating the pituitary gland to secrete ACTH (adrenocorticotropic hormone) (Fig. 1). If there is a deficiency of cortisol, more ACTH is produced, which in turn stimulates the adrenal to produce more cortisol. As a result, more androgens and aldosterone are also produced. A separate pituitary hormone controlling adrenal androgen production has been discovered; however, ACTH is still thought to be the most important modulator of adrenal androgen production. Aldosterone is under a separate control mechanism via the kidney and is only partially affected by ACTH.

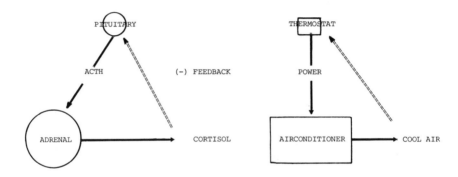

Figure 1. Cortisol levels are monitored by the brain in much the same way as a thermostat works. The brain controls cortisol production by stimulating the pituitary gland to secrete ACTH. The less cortisol, the more ACTH is produced to increase cortisol production.

Physiologic role of the "normal" adrenal and androgen production

At about age 8, the adrenal glands start to increase their production of androgens. While the exact triggering mechanism for this is not known, as has been mentioned, a hormone which specifically turns on adrenal androgen production has been implicated. The role of adrenal androgens would seem to be involved with the onset of sexual maturity. Pubic hair growth and early breast budding are probably the primary result of adrenal androgen production. The elaboration of adrenal androgens may be the signal to the hypothalamus, which results in the changes that cause the onset of puberty. Another function of the adrenal androgens in women may be the protection of the skeleton after menopause. Estrogens promote both calcium absorption from the diet, and the laying down of calcium in bone; loss of estrogens causes rapid bone thinning, or osteoporosis.

The adrenal is the major source of sex steroids in menopausal women. The ovary will continue to produce variable amounts of testosterone for a while, but this will cease with time. These adrenal androgens are converted to estrone, which helps to preserve the skeleton in post-menopausal women.

THE ADRENAL CORTEX AND HIRSUTISM

The key to understanding the role of the adrenal glands in hirsutism is to have some knowledge of the structure and function of the steroid hormones. A hormone is a chemical secreted into the blood stream which causes an effect at a different site in the body. Cells which are responsive to a particular hormone recognize that hormone by means of receptors. The hormone fits the receptor in much the same way as a key fits a lock. The closeness of the fit is termed the affinity of the hormone.

Using the analogy of a blank key cut in different ways by a locksmith to fit many different locks, the basic molecular structure of the adrenal steroids can be considered to be the blank key, and the various steps in the hormone's production may be considered to be teeth cut in the key. If each tooth is cut at a separate factory, each factory may be equated with a step in hormone production, and its workers as an enzyme. Enzymes are responsible for the addition or subtraction of atoms at specific loci of the molecule. The important thing to remember is that while the addition or subtraction of an atom may not seem to change the structure of the molecule appreciably, it can cause a vast difference in function. This difference is due to the receptor, and certain hormone precursors produced along the chain of synthesis may fit the receptor to a lesser or greater degree and thus act as hormones themselves. While certain precursors may have low affinity, if they are present in large quantities, they may cause an effect similar to that of the hormone. The active hormone has a higher affinity and needs to be present in much smaller quantities.

Hormone production by the adrenal glands

The basis for all adrenal steroid hormones is cholesterol. Cholesterol is converted to pregnenolone, the common precursor for mineralocorticoid, glucocorticoid, and androgen pathways. At this point, several different conversions are possible. Some pregnenolone is converted to progesterone (a tooth is cut). Both progesterone and pregnenolone then go through a series of identical steps (factories to form two hormones: dehydroepiandrosterone (DHEA) in the case of pregnenolone; and ∇^4-androstenediol (∇^4A) in the case of progesterone. DHEA can then be either converted to testosterone via a conversion of ∇^4- or ∇^5-androstenediol, or be sulfated to DHEAS (dehydroepiandrosterone sulfate), a weak androgen. ∇^4-androstenediol is converted to testosterone in both the adrenal and periphery of the body.

Several precursors in the androgen pathways are also precursors for the mineralocorticoid and glucocorticoid pathways. Pregnenolone and 17-hydroxypregnenolone are converted to progesterone and 17-hydroxyprogesterone. These form the precursors for cortisol and aldosterone, respectively, and go through a series of identical conversion steps to be transformed into these products (Fig. 2). While the control of the quantity of production of each hormone is to a certain extent independent, any increase in the production of one will affect the others.

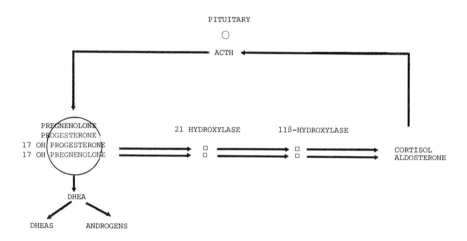

Figure 2.   Normal adrenal pathway.

Adrenal androgens and hirsutism

People vary in their skin sensitivity to androgens as a function of their genetic background. [1, 6] A small increase in circulating androgens, may, therefore, cause a great deal of hirsutism in sensitive individuals. Similarly, a great deal of androgen may be present with little or no hair growth in others. While the adrenal gland does not tend to produce great quantities of androgen, a small increase may produce hirsutism in some individuals.

In certain situations, such as congenital adrenal hyperplasia, Cushing's syndrome, virilizing adrenal tumors, or stress, there may be elaboration of large amounts of adrenal androgens.

Virilizing congenital adrenal hyperplasia

Using our previous analogy of a key production plant, the adrenal hormones go through a number of factories where modifications are made. As previously stated, 17-hydroxyprogesterone and progesterone go through several steps which are identical. What would happen if one of those steps (factories) went on strike?

A strike, as we know, may take the form of a slowdown or a stoppage. If one factory goes on strike, the keys are diverted to other factories and excesses may be produced. This is analogous to a partial or complete enzyme deficiency. As a result of a decrease in production, cortisol levels are lowered. The brain tries to rectify the situation and ACTH production is increased. The amount of precursor to the factories is, therefore, increased to an extent that, in case of a partial enzyme deficiency (slowdown), the pressure may allow the production quotas to be met, and thus cortisol levels may return to normal. The back-up of raw material, however, causes more precursors to go down the remaining unaffected androgen pathway. This pathway is very efficient and an excess of androgens forms.

Two situations exist where this may happen (Figs. 3 and 4). The 21-hydroxylase enzyme and 11-hydroxylase enzyme are two steps in both the cortisol and aldosterone pathways. Total or, more commonly, partial deficiencies of these enzymes occur in families. These are known as the virilizing congenital adrenal hyperplasias. 21-hydroxylase deficiency is responsible for 90% of cases of congenital adrenal hyperplasia. Inheritance is variable; with an inheritor of one gene having a mild form of the disease, and an inheritor of both genes having severe disease, spontaneous cases have been seen. On the other hand, the 11β-hydroxylase deficiency is an autosomal recessive gene and both parents contribute to this disorder.

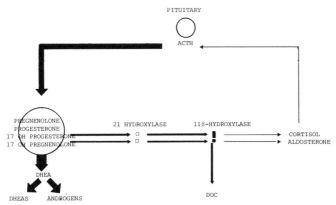

Figure 3. 21-hydroxylase deficiency. Block at 21-hydroxylase causes DHEAS and androgens to increase. Decreased aldosterone production causes salt loss; ACTH increases precursor production in order to normalize cortisol levels.

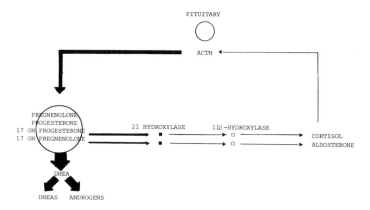

Figure 4. Block at 11β-hydroxylase level. DHEAS and androgens are increased; build-up of desoxycortisol (DOC) causes hypertension; ACTH increases precursor production in order to normalize cortisol levels.

The 21-hydroxylase deficiency occurs earlier in the pathway. Thus, the precursors have no cortisol or aldosterone-like activity and, because aldosterone is the hormone responsible for salt retention, this is called the salt-losing form of congenital adrenal hyperplasia. The 11β-hydroxylase block causes a build-up of a precursor with weak aldosterone activity. Because of the large quantity, however, salt is retained and hypertension may ensue. Thus, this is known as the hypertensive form.

A great deal of excess androgens (DHEA, ∇^4A, and testosterone) may be produced in the complete or near complete blocks. At birth, female babies may be difficult to distinguish from males as the testosterone may masculinize the external genitalia, causing clitoromegaly (Fig. 5), or severe enlargement of the clitoris and fusion of the labia. The excess male hormone will stimulate hair growth in an androgenic pattern in these children, with pubic hair appearing at 3 years of age. The adrenal glands are large due to the excessive stimulation. This appearance led to the term adrenogenital syndrome. Thus, we have the salt-losing and hypertensive forms of the adrenogenital syndrome. Where cortisol is completely absent, death may rapidly ensue. Therefore, it is mandatory that all babies of undetermined sex be evaluated for this disease.

In its milder forms, the androgen excess may be modest. This may lead only to a slight excess of hair in the child. The problem may become manifest at puberty when there is a surge of adrenal activity. While such women do not usually have genital ambiguity, they develop acne and hirsutism and are commonly infertile. Occasionally, the mild form of this syndrome has been described as appearing as late as the third decade of life, with the sudden occurrence of male pattern hair growth and acne.

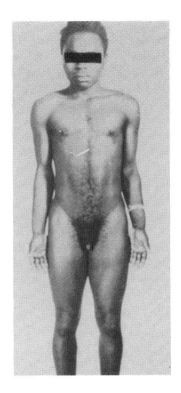

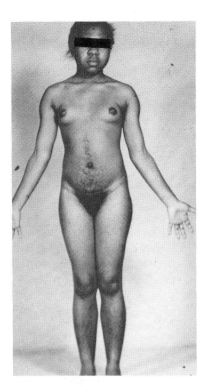

Figure 5. Female patient with congenital adrenal hyperplasia. Note masculine features and enlargement of the clitoris.

Figure 6. Same patient as Fig. 5. Following adequate cortisone therapy, note loss of masculine features and breast development.

Treatment of adrenogenital syndrome

The adrenogenital syndrome, both the 21-hydroxylase and the 11β-dyhdroxylase, are treated with steroid hormone replacement therapy. The patient must be given enough cortisone to completely suppress the ACTH production, and thus prevent the hyperstimulation of the patient's adrenal glands. Adequate treatment in females is essential, as the high levels of adrenal androgens will not only cause distressing side-effects of hirsutism and acne, but it may cause growth retardation in children and also impair the woman's ultimate fertility. With adequate cortisone therapy, breast development and ovulatory menstrual periods may be expected (Fig. 6). Conception often occurs.

Cushing's syndrome

An excess of glucocorticoids as a result of a tumor, Cushing's disease, of the administration of cortico-steroids leads to a distinct appearance. The face becomes rounded (moon facies) because of facial muscle tone and fat deposition on the cheeks (Fig. 7). Fat is deposited on the trunk of the body but not on the limbs, leading to a fat body and skinny arms and legs. A hump of fat forms behind the neck; there is thinning of the skin and easy bruising; and purple striae (stripes) form on the abdomen as a result of stretch marks forming, due to the weight gain and hemorrhage into them. As a result of the excess steroid production, diabetes occurs; decreased calcium absorption and bone formation may lead to fractures; salt retention will lead to high blood pressure. In this condition, two forms of hair growth are noted: vellus hair due to the increased cortisone production; and, in females, the excess androgens will lead to hirsutism and in some cases, virilism.

While this syndrome would appear to be unmistakable, it is not. Many women with polycystic ovaries are also obese and hirsute. Many obese women have high blood pressure and diabetes, and many have stretch marks which may resemble the striae found in Cushing's disease. The diagnosis, therefore, often is not so clearcut, and therefore must be made with care.

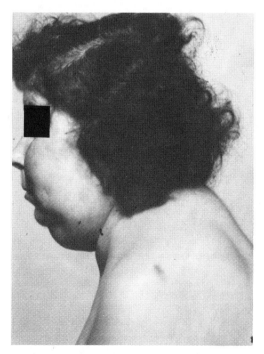

Figure 7.   Patient with Cushing's disease. Note moon shaped face and fat formation of neck.

Cushing's disease

Several situations exist where ACTH levels are increased and lead to an excess of cortisol, androgen, and aldosterone production. Several cancers, especially certain lung and pancreatic cancers, may secrete ACTH. As suspected by Cushing, pituitary adenomas (tumor) secreting ACTH are the most common form of ACTH over-production. Another cause has been thought to be a hypothalamic disorder where the brain may hyperstimulate the pituitary to secrete excess ACTH.

The diagnosis of Cushing's disease can be easily confused with that of polycystic ovarian disease (PCO), when the patient is obese, with or without hirsutism. In PCO, or the adrenal hyperplasias, the gland responds to suppression of morning (8 a.m.) cortisol levels with a low-dose of dexamethasone 1 mg, administered at midnight the night before. A few cases fail to suppress. A 48-hour low-dose test of 0.5 mg of dexamethasone every 6 hours for the 48 hours will cause these few cases to completely suppress cortisone production. Two milligrams (2 mg) of dexamethasone, every 6 hours, will suppress pituitary Cushing's but not tumor-related Cushing's in most cases. Thus, a useful test is available.

The dexamethasone test was originally standardized to urine, with a measurement of 17-hydroxy and 17-ketosteroids. The addition of free cortisol levels, however, in urine testing has added a tremendous degree of sensitivity and specificity to the test. Since 24 hour urines have to be collected, which is often inconvenient, the use of serum cortisol levels has almost as good a sensitivity and specificity, and is much simpler. Invariably, with few exceptions, most non-Cushing's patients will suppress on the overnight dexamethasone suppression; thus, no further testing is needed after this. If the patient suppresses after the low-dose dexamethasone suppression, again no further work-up is believed necessary. If the patient suppresses only after the high-dose dexamethasone suppression test, the pituitary cause of Cushing's should be sought and a computerized x-ray known as a CAT scan of the pituitary should be instituted. This will identify a lesion in the majority of these cases, although an occasional bronchial carcinoma has been known to be responsive to dexamethasone suppression. If the adrenals are still not suppressed after a high dose suppression test, then an adrenal neoplasm or an extra pituitary ACTH producing tumor should be sought. ACTH levels measured at the same time as the high dose suppression test may be useful. If the basal levels of ACTH are suppressed, despite high cortisol levels, an adrenal tumor is likely.

Treatment of Cushing's disease is the treatment of the cause. Removal of the pituitary tumor, where one is identified, is often successful in curing the disease. If the pituitary tumor is not completely removed, pituitary irradiation, and in some rare cases, adrenalectomy may become necessary. Destruction of an ACTH-producing source, such as a carcinoma, is clearly indicated when possible. Removal of an adrenal tumor where it is shown to be causing the Cushing's syndrome is mandatory. Cyproheptadine has been useful as an adjunctive therapy in pituitary Cushing's disease.

Adrenal neoplasms

Adrenal neoplasms are usually small, non-encapsulated masses, and are usually single solitary nodules. However, bilateral zonated nodules have been described, but they probably represent adrenal hyperplasia rather than adenomas, which are small and secrete adrenal steroids independent of ACTH control. The rest of the gland and the contralateral gland are atrophic due to chronic suppression of ACTH by the cortisone production of the tumor.

In contrast, adrenal carcinomas are usually large when discovered and often have metastasized at the time of discovery. It is impossible, however, to distinguish definitely between adrenal adenomas and adrenal carcinomas without histological examination. The diagnosis of adrenal neoplasms is suspected by means of nonsuppressable adrenal hormone production in the presence of high doses of dexamethasone.

Adrenal neoplasms have been reported to occur at vitually any age, from in-utero to old age. However, the average age appears to be 34. The presenting sign in adults is a rapid onset of virilization and Cushing's syndrome. Patients with hirsutism or virilization, resulting from adrenal androgens, will usually have elevated levels of DHEAS. A high testosterone level associated with the normal DHEAS is more likely to be of ovarian origin, whereas a high testosterone associated with a high DHEAS is likely to suggest a tumor of adrenal origin.

Once diagnostic criteria have established a reasonable certainty of an adrenal tumor, radiologic studies should confirm its presence. Studies using a CAT scanner have been very sensitive in identifying adrenal tumors. The presence of an adrenal tumor may be confirmed using angiographic studies and by obtaining blood samples from the adrenal veins. The treatment of adrenal tumors is removal; treatment of adrenal carcinoma, if it is not resectable, is with chemotherapy. The cure rate of benign adrenal tumors should be excellent – approaching 100%. The cure rate for adrenal carcinomas, even with appropriate therapy, is poor, with 75% dying within one year after the diagnosis is made.

Figure 8 a & b is an example of a young virilized woman with an adrenal tumor. The tumor and the kidney were removed in toto. Pathologic exam revealed marked cellular atypia suggesting malignancy (Fig. 9 a & b). After removal of the tumor, much of the hirsutism regressed, menses returned and pregnancy soon ensued (Fig. 10). She has had two children and is alive and well fifteen years after surgery.

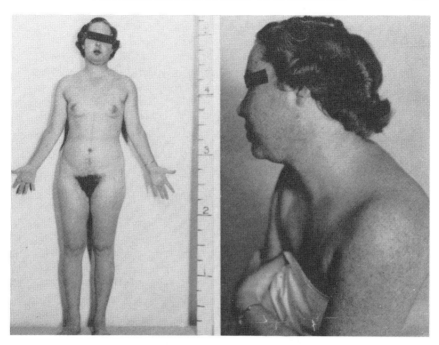

Figure 8.   Virilized patient due to adrenal tumor. Note the round plethoric face, hypertrichosis, acne, striae, and masculine body build. (From Greenblatt, R. B., Scarpa-Smith, C. and Metts, J. C. Fertil Steril 10:323, 1959)

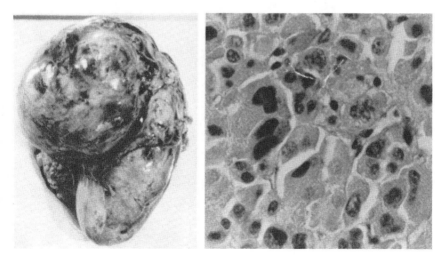

Figure 9.   (a) Adrenal tumor removed from patient shown in Fig. 8   (b) Photomicrograph of a histologic section of the adrenal tumor showing abnormal size and shape of hyperchromatic nuclei. (From: IBID)

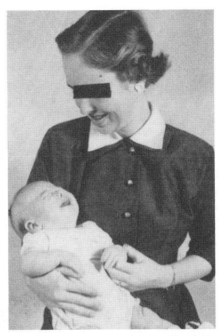

Figure 10. Satisfactory reduction of infertility problem after removal of adrenal tumor.

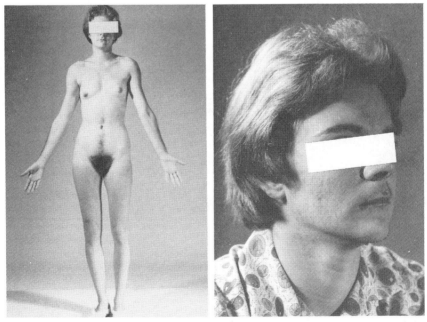

Figure 11. (a) Note the masculine body build with male escutcheon.   (b) Note hairiness of face, chin and upper lip.

Tumors of the adrenal in the female may be solely masculinizing without signs of metabolic upheaval, as in Cushing's syndrome. Such women develop marked hairiness as a rule, increased muscle mass, deep voice, and often increased sex drive. Most become amenorrheic, but some do not. Figure 11 a & b is that of an infertile female who was strongly virilized but continued to menstruate. A benign adrenal tumor was removed and conception soon took place. The hirsutism remained despite removal of the tumor surgery.

Stress

The adrenal gland is the stress gland in the body. Both physical and psychologic stress may increase adrenal-androgen production via an increase in ACTH. Obesity and depression have been shown to cause a defect in the response of the pituitary gland to overnight suppression with a low-dose of dexamethasone. Since obesity and hirsutism frequently co-exist, this could be the operative mechanism for the hirsutism in this situation. This would also seem to incriminate stress as the cause of the increased incidence of hirsutism in psychiatric patients.

As more women enter the job market place, and the stresses involved with modern life are increased, so an increase in adrenal androgens may be expected. It has been chauvinistically stated that competitive women have high male hormone levels, but is this the result and not the cause of their increased ambition?

In order to study the contribution of the adrenal gland to hirsutism, we studied sixty consecutive women with a complaint of hirsutism.[8] A basal testosterone level was drawn on each woman as well as an LH level. In order to standardize the time of the cycle, all samples were taken between the third and ninth days after the onset of menses. The volunteers were then placed on Prednisone 5 mg in the evening, and 2.5 mg in the morning. After two months, blood was again taken for testosterone (T), LH and FSH.

Three groups were observed. Eleven women had a normal baseline testosterone level. Twenty-six women with high testosterone levels had a better than 50% suppression with treatment. Twenty-three women had a worse than 50% suppression of their high T levels. LH and LH:FSH ratios were compared for the groups. Women who had normal testosterone levels had normal LH levels as well. Interestingly, these women suppressed their T levels by nearly 50%. Women who had elevated T levels had elevated LH levels. These women who had a good response suppressed their T levels no differently than the women with normal T levels.

Several points emerge from this study. A significant proportion of women who had hirsutism had normal testosterone levels. This would tend to support the idea of an enhanced skin sensitivity and, doubtless, if this study had been done in a Mediterranean country, the proportion would have been much higher. The fact that these women had a significant reduction in their testosterone levels with low-dose steroid therapy would seem to indicate that this form of therapy may be useful by diminishing the amount of testosterone reaching the skin, even when T levels are normal. Exactly how low a level one would have to achieve in order not to stimulate receptors, however, is yet unknown.

The women in the second group had a marked response and had their T levels drop by a mean of 75%. This is the group of women that we postulate are the adrenal hyperproducers of androgens and would respond best to adrenal suppression. Some of those women, one would suspect, have a mild form of 21- or 11β-hydroxylase deficiency.

The third group of patients, who did not respond to suppression, we assume are predominantly ovarian androgen producers.

ADRENAL EVALUATION OF THE HIRSUTE WOMAN

Any professional consulted about excess hair growth should evaluate the condition. Often a simple history will give many clues to the underlying problem. An examination of the pattern of hair growth is also useful. In addition, an informed electrologist has often been the person to spot the cause of the underlying problem.

Women presenting with hirsutism should be asked about the duration of hair growth. Hair growth which appeared at puberty, but has not changed much since then, is not as significant as a recent onset of hair growth or hair growth which is getting worse. In treating a patient with electrolysis, the failure of electrolysis to control the hair growth, despite frequent visits, should be an alert to an underlying medical condition.

Women should be asked about fertility. The length of the menstrual cycle and duration of menses may be perfectly normal. Only by placing the woman on a temperature chart, or by an endometrial biopsy, may the problem of a defective ovulatory pattern be elicited.

Since irregular menses and amenorrhea tend to occur at higher levels of androgen production, a woman with hirsutism and irregular menses needs a thorough medical evaluation to rule out an adrenal hyperplasia or a tumor of ovarian or adrenal origin.

Family social history is of vital importance. Hirsutism in a woman who gives a history of coming from a hairy, but fertile, family is of less significance than one where the woman is the only one affected. The adrenal hyperplasias are genetically inherited. Mothers and daughters are often both affected, as are other family members. If the patient gives a history of her hirsute mother having had irregular menses or a hysterectomy for abnormal bleeding, this is a suspicious sign for partial 21- or 11β-hydroxylase deficiency.

A hair chart which allocates points for several areas of abnormal distribution is useful since a few hairs in any location, alone, may not be significant, but a combination may lead to suspicion of hyperandrogenism. Finding hair in some areas may, however, be of more significance than others. Terminal chin hair, hair on the chest, or hair above the umbilicus is, in my experience, almost always significant. Using the chart, I allocate points for moustache, hair on the side of face, chin, peri-areolar area, as well as chest, abdomen, buttocks, and peri-anal areas, toes and fingers. Hair on the lower arms and legs may not be androgen-related. A few hairs in an oriental woman or a Caucasian woman with fine hair may be more significant than a Mediterranean woman with luxurious hair growth.

MEDICAL EVALUATION OF HIRSUTISM

After a history and physical, women are placed on a basal body temperature graph. The temperature is taken every morning, before rising, and entered on the graph. Oral temperatures will suffice. The purpose of this graph is to evaluate ovulation to make sure that blood tests are taken in the correct part of the cycle. A normal basal body temperature graph will have a 14 day $\pm$ 2 follicular phase, and a 14 day $\pm$ 2 luteal phase. The temperature, which is low during the follicular phase, will rise by half a degree, or so, during the luteal phase. A luteal phase of 10 days or less may cause one to suspect ovulatory dysfunction.

Serum androgen levels are measured during the early part of the cycle. These measurements include testosterone and DHEAS. Dexamethasone 0.5 mg is then administered every 6 hours for 48 hours, and androgen levels are again obtained. Interpretation of the data obtained may be difficult since most laboratories have not standardized their data to the early part of the cycle; and, testosterone levels may range as high as 1.2 ng/ml during mid-ovulation. My studies have found that the average testosterone level for normal women early in the cycle is around 0.3 ng/ml with an upper range of 0.4 ng/ml, and other studies have confirmed these results. A significant suppression of testosterone levels in a hirsute woman, however, is important because no matter what the testosterone levels are, significantly reducing these levels should help the hirsutism.

DHEAS levels may also be useful since a high DHEAS level would almost certainly implicate the adrenal in the production of the excess androgens. A failure of DHEAS to suppress would lead one to suspect an adrenal tumor. I routinely obtain LH and FSH levels on the baseline blood sample, since an increase in LH:FSH ratio over 2 is commonly associated with hyperandrogenism. A free-testosterone level may be of some use where the total testosterone level is normal.

A new test, now available from Nichols Laboratory, 3-alpha-Diol G (3 α-Androstanediol Glucuronide) is a sensitive test for breakdown products of dihydrotestosterone (DHT). This may give extremely useful information in hirsute women, even when the testosterone levels are normal, since this is a test of skin sensitivity. A significant reduction of 3-alpha-Diol G levels after dexamethasone suppression would show that treatment by adrenal suppression may be extremely useful in the control of hirsutism. Both testosterone and 3-alpha-Diol G must be measured early in the cycle, days 3 to 9, since they can rise sharply, even in normal women, at the time of ovulation. The concurrent use of a temperature chart will help to eliminate false-positive results.

TREATMENT OF HYPERANDROGENISM

Even if hyperandrogenism has been found to be predominantly adrenal, certain cases may occasionally still respond to the birth control pill. However, some hirsute women may get worse, as has been mentioned in the chapter on iatrogenic hirsutism. The progestogens used in the pill are, themselves, androgenic and also may displace the testosterone from its binding globulin, thus increasing the amount available for metabolism. However, in clinical practice this is rarely, if ever, observed.

When androgens are shown to be primarily of adrenal origin, clearly the treatment of choice is adrenal suppression. A low-dose of Prednisone, using 2.5 mg in the morning and 5 mg at night, will suppress the adrenal gland and probably is low enough not to cause any other side effects. After two months of treatment, blood testosterone levels are measured. If they are adequately suppressed, the dose of Prednisone may be cut back to 5 mg/day, administered in the afternoons, and serum androgens again assessed in order to see if the suppression is maintained. Occasionally, women can be weaned off the adrenal suppression with no further rise in their androgen levels.

Where women are desirous of contraception, it may be worthwhile to try them on the birth control pill and again to measure their serum androgen levels. If these are not suppressed by the birth control pill, the combination of adrenal suppression and the birth control pill has been shown to be effective in suppressing androgens.

The drug spironolactone, which is an aldosterone antagonist, also interferes with the production of androgens. It has been shown to be useful as an adjunct to therapy, either with the oral contraceptive or with steroids, or both. It must be remembered that it requires very little androgen to stimulate an established terminal hair, and that the existing hairs are probably going to be maintained, even at low levels of androgens, until they naturally fall out.

Thus, the primary treatment of terminal hair is electrolysis. The hormonal treatment of the condition, however, will slow down new hair growth; thus, the patient becomes controllable with electrolysis therapy.

References

1. Yen SSC: The polycystic ovary syndrome. Clin Endocr 12:177, 1980
2. Jones, G. E. S., Howard, J. E. and Langford, H. The use of cortisone in follicular phase disturbances. Fertil Steril 4:49, 1953
3. Greenblatt, R. B. Cortisone in the treatment of hirsute women. Am J Obstet Gynecol 66:700, 1953
4. Horton, R., Neisler, J. Plasma androgens in patients with polycystic ovary syndrome. J Clin Endocrinol Metab 28:479, 1968
5. Bardin, C. W., Hembree, W. D. and Lipsett, M. D. Suppression of testosterone and androstenedione production rates with dexamethasone in women with idiopathic hirsutism and polycystic ovaries. J Clin Endocrinol Metab 28:1300, 1968
6. Abraham, G. E., Buster, J. E. Peripheral and ovarian steroids in ovarian hyperthecosis. Obstet Gynecol 47:581, 1976
7. Rodriguez-Rigau, L. J., Smith, K. D. and Tcholakian, R. K., et al: Effect of prednisone on plasma testosterone levels and on duration of phases of the menstrual cycle in hyperandrogenic women. Fertil Steril 32:408, 1979
8. Karpas, A. E., Rodriguez-Rigau, L. J., Smith, K. D. and Steinberger, E., Effect of acute and chronic androgen suppression by glucocorticoids on gonadotropin levels in hirsute women. J Clin Endocrinol Metabolism 59, p 780, 1984

9
Sexual Development Disorders Associated with Masculinization at Puberty

Santiago L. Padilla, M.D.
Paul G. McDonough, M.D.

INTRODUCTION

Genetic, anatomic, and endocrine abnormalities of sexual development may be diagnosed at birth, especially if they present with ambiguous genitalia. This is the ideal situation because surgical and medical treatment may be instituted early enough to prevent serious gender identity problems, as well as physical, emotional and sexual handicaps. Regretfully, many of the disorders are either missed at birth because the defects are very subtle and considered "normal variants", or its manifestation does not become evident until puberty with resumption of sex hormone production. At that time sexual development, especially untoward hair growth, may pose a serious problem to an individual with an intersex disorder who has been reared as a female.

Intersex disorders are disorders of sexual differentiation with varying degrees of discordance between the chromosomal sex, the external genital organs, and the secondary sexual characteristics. The specific intersex disorders that may result in abnormal degrees of hair growth or masculinization at puberty are referred to as mixed gonadal dysgenesis, female pseudohermaphroditism, male pseudohermaphroditism, and true hermaphroditism.

PHYSIOLOGY OF SEX DIFFERENTIATION AND PUBERTY

The sex of an individual is determined by genetic, endocrine, anatomic and psychological factors. Normal sexual differentiation involves multiple events beginning with sperm and egg formation, fertilization and early embryonic development, and continues through puberty. Early cellular division is especially important in assuring a normal chromosome number for the embryo.

Fetal sex differentiation, as described by Jost,[1] will occur along female lines unless male differentiation is actively imposed by genetic and/or endocrine factors at critical stages of embryonic development.

Gonadal differentiation

Testicular differentiation is initiated at 4-6 weeks gestation and is dependent upon the presence of testicular determinants located on the Y-chromosome. It appears to be controlled by a substance known as H-Y antigen,[2] and coincides with production of a Mullerian Inhibiting factor (MIF) which will inhibit the development of the vagina, uterus and fallopian tubes. Leydig cells responsible for testosterone production by the testis appear at around 4-6 weeks gestation. In contrast, ovarian differentiation occurs later at 6-8 weeks.

Differentiation of the genital duct system

All human fetuses are endowed with two pairs of internal primitive reproductive system ducts: the Wolffian or mesonephric ducts, and the Mullerian or paramesonephric ducts. Before sexual differentiation starts there is no difference between male and female embryos in these systems.

Male duct system differentiation is mediated by two discrete substances secreted by the testes: (a) testosterone, which guides the Wolffian ducts and the external genitalia along male lines, and (b) Mullerian inhibiting factor, that will inhibit development of the internal female reproductive system.

In the absence of testes, female differentiation will occur; the Wolffian ducts degenerate and the Mullerian ducts will develop into the fallopian tubes, uterus and upper vagina.

Differentiation of external genitalia

The external genitalia of both sexes are identical up to 9 weeks gestation (40 mm stage). Masculinization begins by increasing the anogenital distance. The primitive 'labia' then fuse to form the scrotum. Penile organogenesis is completed by 12-14 weeks (70-90 mm). After this period, labial fusion cannot be obtained in female fetuses by testosterone exposure.[3] Penile growth will continue throughout gestation stimulated by testosterone from the fetal testes.

The masculinizing effect on the external genitalia occurs by binding of the androgen, testosterone, to a receptor in the cytoplasm. Testosterone is converted intracellularly to another androgen, dihydrotestosterone (DHT) by the enzyme 5α-reductase. The intracellular receptor exhibits a higher affinity towards DHT, making it a more potent androgen. The external genitalia develop high 5α-reductase activity at the time of sex differentiation because DHT is indispensable for normal differentiation along male lines.

NORMAL PUBERTAL DEVELOPMENT

Complex endocrine mechanisms, not fully understood yet, control the onset and progression of puberty. Genetic, nutritional, endocrine, physical, psychological and environmental factors may all influence the age at which puberty will occur.

In females, puberty begins with an acceleration of linear growth rate which is followed by breast budding, or thelarche. Appearance of the breast bud occurs between ages of 9 and 11, and represents the first clinical sign of increased ovarian estrogen production. Further breast development follows a predictable pattern described by Tanner.[4] Growth of pubic and axillary hair, also known as adrenarche or pubarche, follows shortly after thelarche except in 15% of adolescents where the sequence is inverted. Menarche, the initiation of menses, occurs between ages 11 and 15, with a mean age of 12.8 years. Although menarche has been considered the culminating event of puberty, it is not until ovulation occurs that the ultimate requirement of puberty is fulfilled, i.e., reproduction.

In males, a modest increase in testicular size is the first sign of puberty and occurs between ages 10 and 12. This is followed by an increase in pigmentation of the scrotum and the appearance of pubic hair. Progression of pubertal development with lengthening and thickening of the penis will follow in close relation to the secretion of testosterone. Although growth kinetics are enhanced from early puberty, maximal velocity occurs at around 15 years of age.

Ovarian and testicular hormone production, responsible for the development of secondary sexual characteristics, are stimulated by the pituitary hormones, follicle stimulating hormone (FSH) and luteinizing hormone (LH).

Hormonal changes precede physical changes of puberty. During the childhood years, both FSH and LH remain suppressed. The first true hormonal manifestation of puberty is the appearance of sleep-related pulses of luteinizing hormone (LH). After this, the first signs of puberty will become evident.

The adrenal gland may also play an important role since the androgens, dehydroepiandrosterone (DHEA) and its sulphate (DHEA-S), which are mainly adrenal in origin, increase as early as 2-3 years prior to the pulsatile LH secretion. Puberty culminates with ovulation in the female and active spermatogenesis in the male, allowing reproduction.

Activation of ovarian or testicular sex hormone production at puberty uncovers abnormalities of sexual development not diagnosed at birth, by causing unexpected feminization or masculinization of the individual.

SYNDROMES OF ABNORMAL SEXUAL DEVELOPMENT

Mixed gonadal dysgenesis

Normal females contain two intact sex chromosomes. Deprivation of sex chromosome material may cause abnormal ovarian differentiation (gonadal dysgenesis). Multiple different chromosomal abnormalities may cause gonadal dysgenesis. In our series, mosaicism (presence of different chromosomal complements secondary to abnormal early embryonic division, i.e., 45,X/46,XY) was the most common karyotype involving 49 individuals (58%).[5] The classical cause of gonadal dysgenesis 45,X, with complete absence of one X chromosome, was present in only 27 subjects (32%).

The most common mosaic was 45,X/46,XY in which, at very early embryonic division, a Y chromosome was lost. This deprivation of Y chromosome material may also cause abnormal gonadal differentiation. The term mixed gonadal dysgenesis has been used for these individuals. Their presentation is variable, but includes otherwise normal females that develop masculinization at puberty.

The clinical spectrum of individuals with mosaic 45,X/46,XY karyotypes includes: non-masculinized classical Turner females (short stature, sexually infantile, webbed neck, low hairline and other anomalies), masculinized Turner females and individuals with overt sexual ambiguity. These subjects will have short stature presumably due to their 45,X cell line and masculinization may occur if Y determinants in the 46,XY cell line are sufficient to produce a testis.

Non-masculinized Turner females: These patients consistently have short stature and sexual infantilism. Other physical Turner stigmata, like webbed neck, shield chest, wide spaced nipples, etc., may or may not be present. Clinical identification of individuals in this group may occur at puberty when they present with delayed sexual development.

In our series, the pathological findings in these non-masculinized 45,X/46,XY females were consistently bilateral intra-abdominal streaks accompanied by normal fallopian tubes.[6]

Masculinized Turner females: These subjects usually present with prepubertal clitoral enlargement which is usually augmented at puberty and accompanied by hirsutism (Fig. 1). The pathologic finding is consistently a unilateral testes and a contralateral streak gonad, both intra-abdominal in location. The streak gonads will uniformly have a fallopian tube in the adnexae. The degree of testicular competence is variable and the adnexal structures on the side of the testes may be a fallopian tube or male accessory organs (i.e., vas deferens). This occurs because Mullerian inhibiting factor production may be inadequate to suppress fallopian tube development. The inadequate androgen production only produces clitoromegaly, and the degree of sexual ambiguity seen with the descended testes group does not occur. At puberty these individuals will masculinize as a consequence of testosterone production by their unilateral intra-abdominal testes.

Sexual ambiguity patients: Unilateral descended testes and a contralateral streak will cause frank sexual ambiguity in these individuals. The descended testis seems to be an effective producer of Mullerian inhibiting factor and testosterone, so the accessory structure usually is a vas deferens.

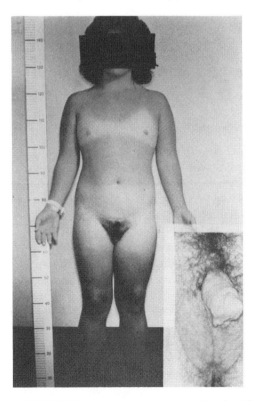

Figure 1. 15-year-old 45,X/46,XY mixed gonadal dysgenesis female with absence of menses, short stature and clitoral enlargement at puberty.

The sex of rearing will depend on the functional capacity of the genitalia. If female gender is selected, the descended testes should be removed to prevent masculinization at puberty, and hormonal supplementation with estrogen should be started at around age 11.

The presence of a Y chromosome predisposes intra-abdominal streaks and testes to the development of germ cell tumors, mainly gonadoblastomas and dysgerminomas, the latter being malignant. The malignant potential dictates the surgical removal of these gonads.

Intersex disorders

A disturbance of the normal process of fetal sexual differentiation may result in malformation or sexual ambiguity. Disorders of sexual differentiation have traditionally been classified into three categories according to gonadal morphology. *Female pseudohermaphroditism* describes abnormal masculinization of the 46,XX fetus. *Male pseudohermaphroditism* is the result of incomplete virilization of the 46,XY fetus. The *true hermaphrodite* is an individual that has both ovarian and testicular tissue irrespective of the karyotype. Extreme caution has to be used to avoid utilization of these terms in front of the patient or their family because of the obvious social implications. Phrases like "your body is male on the outside but female on the inside" should be condemned.

Male pseudohermaphrodites

Causes of male pseudohermaphroditism will include (a) inborn errors of testosterone synthesis; (b) 5α-reductase deficiency; and (c) incomplete androgen sensitivity.

a.   *Inborn errors of testosterone synthesis:* Figure 2 illustrates normal steroid synthesis. The most common affected enzymes are 3 β-hydroxysteroid dehydrogenase (No. 1) and 17 β-ketoreductase (No. 6). These disorders occur as recessively inherited conditions and, in some, both the testes and the adrenal cortex are affected, leading to incomplete adrenal hyperplasia. Most of these defects are rare and have a high mortality.

1. *3 β-hydroxysteroid dehydrogenase deficiency:* Severe salt loss accounts for a high mortality in infancy, but some subjects have survived to puberty, which has been characterized by virilization and breast development (gynecomastia).

2. *17 β-ketoreductase:* This enzyme converts androstenedione to testosterone and estrone to estradiol. The typical features are a partially masculinized male at birth with further virilization at puberty and occasional gynecomastia.

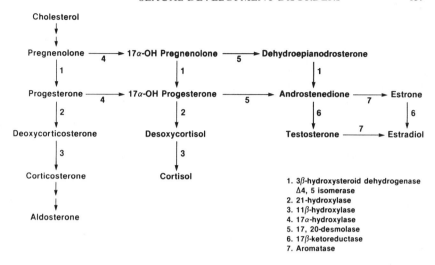

Figure 2. Steroid biosynthesis.

b. *5 α-reductase deficiency:* Testosterone is converted intracellularly to dihydrotestosterone (DHT) by the enzyme 5 α-reductase. DHT binds to an intracellular receptor protein and is transported to the nucleus to initiate protein synthesis. Deficiency of 5 α-reductase impairs conversion of testosterone to DHT, the androgen responsible for masculinization of the external genitalia. Affected persons are 46,XY males, characterized by a female external genitalia at birth, the presence of bilateral testes and normal accessory male structures. At puberty there is virilization of the external genitalia with pubic and axillary hair growth, without gynecomastia. This latter event may be due to higher testosterone levels at puberty than during embryogenesis.

Deficiency of 5 α-reductase is diagnosed by an elevated plasma ratio of testosterone to DHT. Serial administration of human chorionic gonadotropin (HCG), which stimulates testicular production of testosterone, will further elevate the ratio and confirm the diagnosis. Other terms applied to this condition are: Pseudovaginal perineoscrotal hypospadias and 'familial incomplete male pseudohermaphroditism type 2'. If affected persons are to be reared as females, castration should be done before puberty to prevent the virilizing effects of the testes. Estrogen substitution should be started around age 11. If sex of rearing is male, then repair of the hypospadias and revision of the external genitalia should be performed before the child starts to attend school.

c. *Incomplete androgen sensitivity:* These individuals have normal testosterone production and a partial degree of deficient end-organ receptors, thereby causing incomplete masculinization of the external genitalia. At puberty, some virilization occurs and is usually associated with gynecomastia. A wide clinical spectrum occurs with some patients having a predominant female appearance (Lub's syndrome) and others more masculinized with perineal hypospadias (Reifenstein's syndrome). Wilson et al.[7] reported 11 subjects with this condition inherited as an X-linked recessive trait, and suggested grouping these patients under the term 'familial incomplete male pseudohermaphroditism type 1'. Removal of the gonads is necessary if sex of rearing is female to prevent masculinization at puberty.

Female Pseudohermaphrodites

Female pseudohermaphrodites have 46,XX karyotypes with normal ovaries, fallopian tubes, uterus and vagina, but virilized external genitalia. The principle causes of female pseudohermaphroditism are listed in Table 1.

Table 1. Causes of Female Pseudohermaphroditism

A. Exessive fetal androgen production
  1. 21-hydroxylase enzyme deficiency
  2. 11β-hydroxylase enzyme deficiency
  3. 3β-hydroxysteroid dehydrogenase enzyme deficiency
B. Fetal exposure to maternal androgens
C. Unexplained

Congenital adrenal hyperplasia (CAH) secondary to a number of enzymatic deficiencies is the most common cause. Deficient cortisol production causes increased ACTH secretion, therefore stimulating further androgen production. The degree of virilization may range from minimal clitoral enlargement and mild labial fusion to a normal penile development. Lack of descended gonads is the only consistent finding.

The most common enzyme deficiency is 21-hydroxylase followed by 11 β-hydroxylase and 3 β-hydroxysteroid dehydrogenase (Fig. 2).[8] Even though the CAH patient is usually diagnosed at birth, especially because these babies may be salt-losers, some of these children are not diagnosed until later when further masculinization, growth and premature epiphyseal closure occurs. The excessive androgen production can be controlled by inhibiting ACTH with corticosteroids. These patients, if treated properly, may be fertile.

An 'adult onset' and a 'cryptic form' of 21-hydroxylase deficiency have also been identified. This condition, inherited in an autosomal recessive fashion, will usually present with anovulation, amenorrhea, and varying degrees of hirsutism and/or virilization at puberty or after puberty (Fig. 3). The diagnosis is usually made by elevated androgen levels and an exaggerated response of 17α-OH progesterone (which is the enzyme's substrate) after ACTH stimulation. It may be easily confused with other causes of amenorrhea and hirsutism, especially polycystic ovarian disease (PCO).

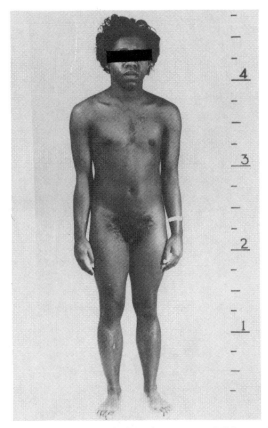

Figure 3. 18-year-old female with 21-hydroxylase enzyme deficiency who presents with absence of menses and virilization at puberty.

Appropriate management with corticosteroids may have excellent response with frequent resumption of ovulation, and cessation of further abnormal hair growth and virilization.

True hermaphrodites

The diagnosis of true hermaphroditism is made when both ovarian stroma with follicles and testicular tissue with distinct tubules are present. The first true hermaphrodite in the medical literature was described by Salen in 1899.[9] True hermaphrodites are classified by their gonadal distribution. An ovary on one side with a contralateral testis, or an ovotestis on one side with a contralateral ovary are the most common combinations. Bilateral ovotestis or alternating ovotestis and testis can also be found.

Clinical presentation: Before puberty the most common presenting symptom is sexual ambiguity. After puberty, the development of gynecomastia and/or menses in a patient reared as a male is a frequent reason for seeking medical advice (Fig. 4). Masculinization, inguinal hernias or absence of menses were common reasons for referral of patients reared as females.

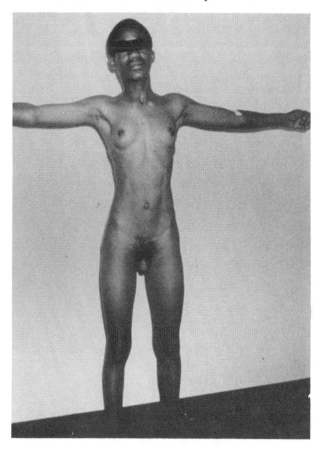

Figure 4.   15-year-old 46,XX true hermaphrodite, reared as a male, with gynecomastia at puberty.

Six families with two or three affected siblings have been reported, suggesting autosomal recessive inheritance.

Clinical findings: Sex of rearing is usually male but the habitus is feminized at puberty, especially because 70% or more of these individuals will develop gynecomastia. A phallus is usually present, with a single opening at the base of the phallus with both urethra and vagina emptying into it. Labioscrotal folds were variable from normal scrotum all the way to normal labia.

Careful palpation of the labioscrotal folds and inguinal canal for presence of gonads is extremely important in evaluating the intersex patient because only gonads with testicular tissue (i.e., testes or ovotestis) will descend. A gonad in the labioscrotal pouch will rule out female pseudohermaphroditism.

The most common karyotype of true hermaphrodites is 46,XX (58.2%) followed by 46,XX/46,XY (13.4%) and 46,XY (11.6%). Gonadal and peripheral blood karyotype are usually concordant.

Gonadal tumours: Germ cell tumors have been found in these patients including dysgerminomas, seminoma, embryonal carcinoma and gonadoblastoma. The overall incidence is thought to be 2.6%. Presence of a 'Y' chromosome has been associated with these tumors, even though we have reported a gonadoblastoma on a true hermaphrodite with a 46,XX karyotype.

MANAGEMENT OF SEXUAL DEVELOPMENT DISORDERS

The most important aspect of management of these individuals is making the appropriate diagnosis at birth and establishing sex of rearing. The decision of sex of rearing should be made in consultation with the parents and according to the functional ability of the external genitalia. In many instances, it will be found advisable to rear the patient as female because an adequate and functional vagina would be easier to establish than an adequate penis.

If sex of rearing is female, feminizing surgery (clitoroplasty and revision of genitalia) should be performed before the child is discharged to prevent embarassment when encountering the rest of the family and friends. If sex of rearing is male, then the genitalia should be repaired to make the penis look normal and if possible a penile urethra constructed by the time the child starts school.

Gonadal preservation will also depend on sex of rearing and position of the gonad. All intra-abdominal gonads in the presence of a Y chromosome should be removed to prevent tumor formation. If female sex of rearing is selected, then all testicular tissue should be removed to prevent masculinization at puberty. On the other hand, if male sex of rearing is selected, then ovarian tissue needs to be removed to prevent gynecomastia at puberty.

If the diagnosis is encountered at or after puberty, then gender role and identity, as well as sex of rearing and functional capacity of the genitalia, need to be evaluated extremely carefully. Certainly at this time the decision is not as easy as at birth and the consequences may be much more serious for the affected individual. The concept that, "once established, gender identity and role are more or less fixed" has now been questioned. Although change of gender may be difficult, the possibility of conversion should be viewed with an open mind in the individual who, because of hormonally induced masculinization or feminization at puberty, finds existance in the original gender intolerable.

SUMMARY

Masculinization at puberty is clearly a result of increased androgen production. The sources of androgens are either ovarian, adrenal, or neoplastic. A careful medical history, family history, and physical examination has to be carried out. Special attention is needed for Turner's syndrome stigmata, gynecomastia, hypospadias, ambiguous genitalia, presence of a vagina, cervix and uterus. A careful examination for the presence of gonads in the labioscrotal pouch or inguinal canal, as well as pelvic or abdominal masses is imperative. Appropriate endocrine, chromosomal, and radiological studies then need to be ordered according to the clinical presentation of each case.

Ideally, the diagnosis of abnormalities of sexual development should be done at birth, so that medical and surgical treatments can be initiated immediately and prevent social, emotional and physical consequences. The diagnosis sometimes is not made until puberty or after puberty when gonadal sex steroid production, stimulated by gonadotropins, causes feminization or masculinization.

Mistakes committed either by the physician, the medical staff, or the family may cause gender identity problems as well as unnecessary physical, emotional and sexual handicaps for the individual.

Objective informed consent with all the implications of management versus no management is imperative. In the best interest of the patient, prompt treatment, carefully adjusted for each individual, should be started as soon as the diagnosis is made, regardless of the age.

References

1. Jost, A., A new look at the mechanism controlling sex differentiation in mammals. Johns Hopkins Med J 130:38, 1972
2. Wachtel, S. S., *H-Y Antigen in the Biology of Sex Determination*. New York, Grune and Stratton, 1983
3. Grumback, M. M. and Durcharme, J. R., The effects of androgens on fetal sexual development, androgen induced female pseudohermaphroditism. Fertil Steril 11:157, 1960
4. Tanner, J. M., Growth and Endocrinology of the Adolescent. In, *Endocrine and Genetic Diseases of Childhood*, Garner, L. I., (ed). Philadelphia, S. B. Saunders, 1969, pp 19-69

5. Butler, W. J., McDonough, P. G. and Huffman, J. W., The spectrum of gonadal dysgenesis. Contemp OB/GYN 23:57, 1983
6. McDonough, P. G. and Tho S. P., The spectrum of 45,X/46,XY gonadal dysgenesis and its applications. Pediatr Adolescent Gynecol 1:1, 1983
7. Wilson, J. D., Harrod, M J. and Goldstein, J. L., et al, Familial incomplete male pseudohermaphroditism, Type 1, N Engl J Med 20:1097, 1974
8. New, M. I. and Levin, L. S. Congenital adrenal hyperplasia. Clin Biochem 14:258, 1981
9. Salen, E., Ein fall von hermaphrotismus verus beim menschen. Verh dt Ges Path 2:241, 1899

10
Hormonal Therapy

R. Don Gambrell, Jr., M.D.

Since abnormal hair growth is either stimulated by excess hormone production or is related to follicle sensitivity to androgens, the most effective treatment is based upon decreasing blood levels of testosterone and/or minimizing the biologic activity of androgens with hormone therapy. Surgical treatment is rarely indicated, except in those infrequent cases caused by ovarian or adrenal tumors. Even genetic or familial hirsutism can often be helped with an adjustment of hormones. Acne, frequently associated with hirsutism or secondary to hyperandrogenism, can usually be improved, even in normal hormone states, by suppression of either elevated or normal androgen levels. By decreasing the biologic effect of circulating androgens with estrogen therapy, both hirsutism and acne may be alleviated, if not cured. Other medications work with the estrogens to diminish the effect of androgens at either the hair follicle or sebaceous glands.

ESTROGEN AND/OR PROGESTOGEN THERAPY

The most effective therapy for arresting the progression of hirsutism is estrogens combined with cyclic progestogens. Administration may be by the subcutaneous implantation of estradiol pellets, or by employing moderate dosages or oral estrogens.

Estradiol pellets are preferred since estradiol is the principal human estrogen.[1] This method of therapy is not only effective but is also quite safe and side effects are minimal. Usually, four 25 mg pellets of estradiol are subcutaneously implanted beneath the skin every six months. Moderate blood levels of estradiol are obtained by daily absorption of minute amounts of estradiol from the pellets. Serum gonadotrophins, specifically FSH and LH, are lowered in the blood stream, which in effect puts the ovaries to rest and diminishes serum testosterone levels, as well as levels of other ovarian androgens such as androstenedione. An additional beneficial effect of estrogen therapy is the increased binding of testosterone to binding proteins in the blood, so that much of the circulating androgens become biologically less active. Therefore, even when the source of excessive androgen is from the adrenal, estrogen therapy effectively increases binding of testosterone to the binding proteins and reduces the biologic activity of those androgens.

Oral estrogens do not have the advantage of being the principal human estrogen, but may be just as effective as estradiol pellets though they may involve slightly more side effects. Comparable oral dosages include conjugated estrogens (Premarin) 2.5 to 3.75 mg daily, or ethinyl estradiol (Estinyl) 0.03 to 0.04 mg daily (Table 1). When oral estrogens are used, natural hormones, such as conjugated estrogens, are preferred because of potentially fewer side effects and an effect on the liver. Another natural estrogen, micronized estradiol (Estrace) 2 to 4 mg may be used. Oral estrogens should be prescribed cyclically from day 1 to day 25 of the menstrual cycle to minimize side effects, but they can be given continuously. Their mechanism of action would be the same as for estradiol pellets.

To the estrogen pellet therapy should be added a cyclic progestogen, such as medroxyprogesterone acetate (Provera) 10 mg, or norethindrone acetate (Aygestin or Norlutate) 5 mg for 10 days each month, of each menstrual cycle, from cycle day 16 through 25. The primary purpose for adding the cyclic progestogen is to induce regular menstrual periods or to restore cyclic menses to shed the endometrium (lining of the uterus) and prevent possible development of endometrial hyperplasia.

Theoretically, the more natural progestogens, such as Provera, are preferrable in treatment of hirsutism because Aygestin and Norlutate are derived from testosterone and have some weak androgen activity. However, in actual practice, no problem with stimulating more hair growth has been encountered with these agents. In addition to ensuring regular cyclic menses, progestogen hormones are good gonadotropin suppressors and may actually enhance the suppression aspect of the estrogen therapy.

When estrogens cannot be tolerated, or are not desired by the patient, intramuscular injections of Depo-Provera 150 mg every three months is a reasonable alternative. Oral Provera can also be given in dosages of 30 mg daily, which will alleviate some of the problems associated with hirsutism. Progestogens act primarily as gonadotropin inhibitors but may also decrease ACTH secretion, thus lowering the output of adrenal androgens.

Side effects from the combination estrogen–progestogen therapy are infrequent; however, some women may experience a slight increase in breast size and/or tenderness, which usually abates with time. Abdominal bloating, or a sense of heaviness in the pelvis, may occur during the days on progestogens as

Table 1. Estrogens and Progestogens Available to Treat Hirsutism

Brand Name	Estrogen	Dosage	Brand Name	Progestogen	Dosage
Estrapel Progynon	Estradiol	25 mg/	Provera Curretabs Amen	Medroxyprogesterone Acetate	2.5 mg 10 mg
Premarin Estratab Evex	Conjugated Estrogens Estrified Estrogens Estrified Estrogens	0.625 mg 1.25 mg 2.5 mg	Depo-Provera	Medroxyprogesterone Acetate	100 mg/ml
Estrace	Micronized Estradiol	1 mg 2 mg	Aygestin Norlutate	Norethindrone Acetate	5 mg
Estinyl	Ethinyl Estradiol	0.02 mg	Norlutin	Norethindrone	5 mg
Ogen	Estrone Piperazine	0.625 mg 1.25 mg 2.5 mg 5.0 mg	Megace	Megestrol Estradiol	20 mg 40 mg

the menstrual period is approached. These symptoms can usually be alleviated with the addition of a mild diuretic, such as hydrochlorthiazide 25-50 mg daily, or spironolactone 25 mg twice daily, for seven to 10 days before the period. If these side effects persist, in spite of diuretic therapy, a change to another oral progestogen will help, or progesterone vaginal suppositories 25 mg daily can be substituted for cycle days 16-25.

ORAL CONTRACEPTIVES

Birth control pills are quite effective in treating hirsutism and are taken in the same manner as for contraception: 21 days of pill use followed by seven days without medication.[2] When used to treat hirsutism, moderate dosage estrogen pills should be employed, i.e., those containing 35-40 μg of estrogen, although some patients will respond to lower dosage pills (Table 2). Other patients may require the high dosage contraceptives to retard progression of hirsutism and lower testosterone blood levels.

Androgen production in hirsute women is usually more dependent on the gonadotropin LH than it is on FSH. Suppression of ovarian hormones depends upon adequate suppression of LH. The progestogens in the birth control pills are effective in suppressing LH production by the pituitary so that testosterone, as well as the weaker androgen, androstenedione, production by the ovaries is decreased. In addition to the inhibitory action of the progestational component, further benefit is achieved by an increase in the protein binding hormones induced by the estrogen component in the pill. This increase in the binding proteins in the blood results in a greater binding capacity with a decrease in free testosterone levels. However, it may take up to six months of treatment with birth control pills to decrease testosterone values in hirsute women.

It should be noted that there is a slow response to treatment with either the pellet method of estrogen-progestogen therapy or treatment with oral contraceptives. Patients should be cautioned that therapy will be necessary for at least six months to one year before an observable diminution in hair growth occurs. Furthermore, combined treatment with electrolysis or other depilatory measures is not recommended until hormone suppression therapy has been administered for at least six months. It should also be emphasized that existing hairs will not go away with hormonal suppressive therapy alone. The goal of such therapy is to arrest the progression of hirsutism so that ancillary methods of hair removal will be effective. Hair follicles will no longer be stimulated to grow hair, but growth which has been previously established will not disappear with hormone treatment alone. Some patients return after a period of treatment expressing disappointment because hirsutism is still present. The combination of ovarian suppression to prevent new

Table 2. Comparison of Moderate and High Dosage Oral Contraceptives

| | Ethinyl Estradiol* | | | Mestranol** | |
Brand Name	Dosage	Progestogen	Brand Name	Dosage	Progestogen
Demulen 1/35	35 µg	Ethynodiol 1 mg Diacetate	Enovid-E	100 µg	Norethynodrel 2.5 mg
Demulen	50 µg	Ethynodiol 1 mg Diacetate	Enovid-5mg	75 µg	Norethynodrel 5 mg
Norinyl 1+35	35 µg	Norethindrone 1 mg	Norinyl 1+80	80 µg	Norethindrone 1 mg
Norlestrin 1/50	50 µg	Norethindrone 1 mg Acetate	Norinyl 2mg	100 µg	Norethindrone 2mg
Ortho-Novum1/35	35 µg	Norethindrone1mg	Ortho-Novum1/80	80 µg	Norethindrone 1mg
Ortho-Novum10/11		Norethindrone 0.5-1 mg	Ortho-Novum 2mg	100 µg	Norethindrone 2mg
Ovcon-35	35 µg	Norethindrone 0.4 mg	Ovulen	100 µg	Ethynodiol 1mg Diacetate
Ovral	50 µg	Norgestrel 0.5 mg			

* Moderate dosage oral contraceptive
**High dosage oral contraceptive

hair growth, and electrolysis to remove the established hairs, yields the most complete and effective treatment of hirsutism.

Therapy should be continued for two to three years and then discontinued to observe the patient for a return of ovulation. Following such a period of treatment, the progression of hirsutism is usually arrested for several months to several years. Should abnormal hair growth reoccur, treatment with either estrogen pellets or oral contraceptives can always be reinstituted.

ADRENAL SUPPRESSION

As noted elsewhere in this book, the adrenal is a major contributor to the hyperandrogenic state. When the work-up for hirsutism has identified the adrenals as the principal source of excess androgens, treatment with an adrenal suppressing hormone such as dexamethasone 0.5 mg daily should begin. Even when the adrenal is a principal contributor to elevated androgens, either estrogen-progestogen therapy or oral contraceptive may still be effective in treating the resulting hirsutism. As shown earlier, estrogens increase the binding proteins in the blood stream so that adrenal androgens also become biologically less active. In addition, progestogens may compete with adrenal hormones for receptors, thus lowering levels of ACTH, the pituitary hormone that stimulates the adrenal. Estrogens also increase the binding of cortisol, the principal adrenal hormone, to the binding proteins that transport it. This increases the bound (inactive) cortisol in the blood with a concomitant lowering of ACTH.

In the patient with persistent and progressive hirsutism, after six or more months on either estrogen-progestogen therapy or birth control pills, measurement of dehydroepiandrosterone sulfate (DHEAS), which is primarily an adrenal androgen, should be done. If this androgen level is still elevated above normal, dexamethasone 0.5 mg daily should be added to both the combination estrogen-progestogen therapy and the oral contraceptive treatment. When dexamethasone is used alone in anovulatory women with progressive hirsutism, ovulatory cycles may be induced and the androgen levels in the blood are usually lowered.

BROMOCRIPTINE

Bromocriptine, marketed as Parlodel, is usually reserved for elevated prolactin states and galactorrhea (milk in the breasts) that is frequently associated with hyperprolactinemia. However, some patients with the amenorrhea-galactorrhea syndromes may also develop progressive hirsutism. When prolactin levels are elevated, bromocriptine 2.5 mg twice to thrice daily is the treatment of choice.[3] Ovulation has been induced with bromocriptine in patients with polycistic ovaries without any elevation of prolactin. Bromo-criptine may also be effective in retarding the progression of hirsutism in certain anovulatory states, such as the polycystic ovary syndrome. However, clomiphene citrate remains the treatment of choice when ovulation induction is desired. Unfortunately, clomiphene is of no value in treating hirsutism since it is an indirect ovarian stimulator and may therefore temporarily increase the output of ovarian androgens.

NEW THERAPEUTIC APPROACHES

Until recently, the best therapy that could be offered was hormonal suppression of excess androgens to arrest the progression of hirsutism. Hair already present usually did not regress and adjunctive measures such as electrolysis were necessary for hair removal. During the last three years, however, two medications, spironolactone and cimetidine, have become available in the United States that will actually produce regression of pre-existing hair in some women (Table 3). Another agent, cyproterone acetate, has been widely used in Europe for over a decade to treat hirsutism, but is as yet not available in the United States.

Table 3.   Agents that May Reverse Hirsutism

Generic Name	Brand Name	Dosage
Spironolactone	Aldactone	25 mg 4 times/day
Cimetidine	Tagamet	300 mg 5 times/day
Cyproterone Acetate	Not available in the U.S.	50-100 mg/day

Probably the most effective of these new therapies is spironolactone, which is an aldosterone antagonist.[4] Aldosterone is an adrenal hormone that helps to regulate salt and fluid metabolism but is not related to hirsutism. However, spironolactone has other actions that may be very helpful in causing abnormal hair to regress, but, fortunately, it does not have any adverse effects on normal hair. Spironolactone is thought to have two different actions: (1) partially inhibiting the ovarian production of androgens, and (2) competing for the androgen receptor in the hair follicle. Fortunately, it has no adverse effect on adrenal function and the only known side effect is a diuresis in the first few days of use.

Spironolactone is prescribed in dosages of 25 mg, four times a day, and may be effective when used alone in milder cases of nonprogressive hirsutism, or even in idiopathic or familial hirsutism. Like estrogen-progestogen and oral contraceptive therapy it may take up to six months before any appreciable regression of hair becomes noticeable. Unfortunately, not all patients respond to spironolactone, but at least a three month trial should be given before it is discontinued.

Spironolactone works best as an adjunct to estrogen-progestogen or oral contraceptive therapy. It may even be effective in some women with iatrogenic hirsutism. Patients being treated with androgens do not lose the androgen benefits when spironolactone is added, so they may continue that therapy and yet get less unwanted hair.

Another recent discovery is that cimitidine, a widely used drug for the treatment of stomach ulcers, may also cause regression of hirsutism.[5] As a histamine H_2 receptor antagonist, cimetidine has no known hormonal activity and does not lower androgen levels in the blood. It is thought to function as a peripheral blocker at the receptor level in the hair follicle. Specifically, it blocks the conversion of testosterone to dihydrotestosterone, which is the most potent androgen stimulant of the hair follicle. Cimetidine 300 mg is prescribed five times a day and, like spironolactone, is most effective when used as an adjunct to androgen suppressive therapy with either the estrogen-progestogen or birth control pills. Cimetidine has no known serious side effects but is somewhat expensive. Because it is probably not quite as effective as spironolactone, the latter agent should be used first.

Cyproterone acetate is an antiandrogen with strong progestational properties that has been used extensively in Europe to treat hirsutism for over a decade.[6] It has multiple actions: it is a powerful gonadotrophin inhibitor, markedly reduces ovarian function including decreased androgen and estrogen levels in the blood, and has some adrenal hormone activity that also suppresses ACTH from the pituitary. Glowing reports from Europe indicate that it is very effective in reversing hirsutism, but it will not be available in the U.S. until approval has been granted by the Food and Drug Administration, presumably because of significant side effects. With the high dosages necessary (100 mg) to achieve good results, fatigue and loss of libido are seen, as are such tedious side effects as delayed menstrual periods and breakthrough bleeding.

SUMMARY

Natural estrogen therapy using estradiol pellets combined with a cyclic progestogen is the most effective method for arresting the progression of hirsutism. Progestogens alone may also be used, and moderate dosage oral contraceptives are very effective. It takes up to six months of hormonal suppressive therapy to stop hair follicles from growing new hairs, but adjunctive measures of hair growth control, such as electrolysis, should be delayed until the hirsutism ceases to progress. Patients should be treated for two or three years, but should hirsutism reoccur after cessation of therapy, hormonal suppressive therapy can be re-instituted. For the first time, new adjunctive therapy such as spironolactone and cimitidine are now available to produce regression of pre-existing hair growth.

References

1. Gambrell, R. D., Jr, Regression of polycystic ovaries by estrogen therapy. Obstet Gynecol 47:569, 1976
2. Givens, J. R., Role of oral contraceptives in the treatment of hyperandrogenism of hirsute women. In, *Hirsutism and Virilism*, Mahesh, V. B. and Greenblatt, R. B. (eds). Boston, John Wright, PSG Inc, 1983, pp 351-367
3. Corenblum, B., Hyperprolactinemic polycystic ovary syndrome. IBID, pp 239-246
4. Cumming, D. C., Yang, Y. C. and Rebar, R. W., et al, Treatment of hirsutism with spironolactone. JAMA 247:1295, 1982
5. Vigersby, R. A., Mehlman, I. and Glass, A. R., et al, Treatment of hirsute women with cimetidine. N Engl J Med 303:1042, 1980
6. Gaspand, U. J., Role of antiandrogens in the treatment of acne. In, *Hirsutism and Virilism*, Mahesh, V. B., Greenblatt, R. B., (eds). Boston, John Wright, PSG Inc, 1983, pp 369-394

11
The Symbolism of Hair: For Good and Evil

Wendy Cooper

From earliest time, hair – its length, texture, color, growth, loss – has exerted a strange fascination on mankind. It has inspired passionate outpourings of romantic poetry and prose, and has been woven into our myths and magic, folklore, and legend.

It is a very ancient belief that a hairy man is a virile man, which may even go back to ancestral man whose epigamic hair could win him sexual dominance. Virility and fertility are, popularly if not medically, closely associated, and the seemingly magical power of hair to regenerate itself also reinforced the hair-fertility link. Even today, primitive peoples who have never heard of a hormone are perfectly able to mark, appreciate and use in their customs, magic and folklore, the clear and visible connection between body hair and sexual maturity. In many cultures, by what psychologists would now term 'displacement', the same role has been assigned to head hair. So, throughout the ages, hair has played an important role not only in puberty rites but also in rituals designed to propitiate the gods and ensure fertility in humans, crops, or animals.

The belief in a connection between hair and strength extended, of course, to the beard, often regarded as a sacred token of strength and virility. Jewish Elders imposed a strict law forbidding the shaving "of the four corners of the face", which is still observed by strict Orthodox Jews. In ancient Babylon, beards were held in such esteem that oaths were sworn upon them, and throughout history, in many cultures, to pull a man's beard was an assault upon his honor.

Shaving the hair of a defeated enemy was a common humiliation and one imposed by Rome on both the hairy Gaul and the almost equally hairy Briton, who, although beardless, wore long hair and long moustaches. Punishment involving forcible shaving or cropping has, of course, sexual implications. Because of the links between pubic hair and the genitals, and by 'displacement' between head hair and sexual power, the cutting off of a man's hair is a symbolic castration. Hindu culture recognizes this; a Brahmin, for example, wears the tonsoured tuft to represent sexual restraint, a shaven head for celibacy, or matted hair for total detachment from the sexual passions. In Buddhist Sri Lanka, there is a similar distinction: celibate monks have their heads shaved. This may be seen as a sign that they do not exercise their virility and are sexual non-combatants.

With women, too, hair is such an explicit expression of sexuality that even today some Orthodox Jewish women crop their hair at marriage, and afterwards conceal their natural hair from the sight of everyone but their husband. Concealment is often a substitute for cutting off the hair, and so Catholic nuns cover their hair with a coif. Arabs long considered it more shameful for a married woman to be seen with her hair uncovered than to be seen naked.

In very recent times in liberated France toward the end of World War II, women suspected of consorting with the occupying German troops had their heads publicly shaved. This was a punishment and humiliation; but it also represented removing the loose hair of promiscuity, with head shaving a substitute not for castration so much as for rape.

Though hair in both sexes is symbolic of sexuality, deep down in atavistic memory the link between hair and strength survives. With it until this more prosaic age, also survived the belief in the spiritual. In the Isle of Skye off Scotland, 'grugach', meaning hairy, is still used today as a name for the sun.

Solar hair was often depicted as seven distinct locks or rays, a number which may have had planetary significance in those days. Certainly, numerous representations of sun-gods from widely different cultures used this idea.

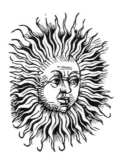 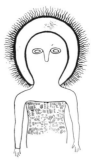

Figure 1. The face of the sun, seen as a human head with hair forming the sun's life-giving rays (left). An Australian cave painting which probably also represents a sun-god. (From: Cooper, W., *Hair: Sex, Society Symbolism.* New York Stein and Day/Publishers, 1971)

A Pompeian wall painting shows Helios with his head encircled with seven well-defined rays; the Persian sun-god Mithras, in addition to abundant hair, had seven beams like hairy spikes. Even early Christian art sometimes showed the figure of Christ with seven solar rays around his head, and a stylized version of this came to form the halo, converting in the temporal sphere to the crown as a symbol of sovereignty and power.

So hair acquired its touch of divinity in an ancient space shuttle from man to gods and back to man, becoming a symbol of the magical and spiritual power of the gods. And always, the solar heroes who emerged over the ages, part mythical and part historical figures, possessed splendid heads of hair, along with enormous physical strength, sexual prowess and magical power – yet all of this waned if the hair was cut.

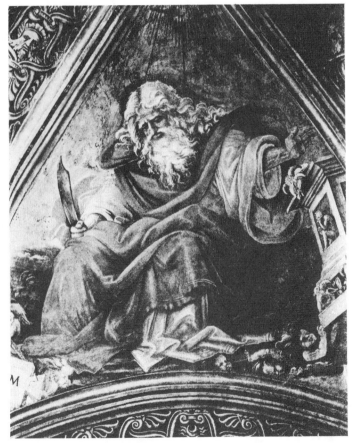

Figure 2.   The prophet Abraham, from the fresco by Filippino Lippi (c. 1457-1504) in the Church of S. Maria Novella in Rome. Although artists tended to portray biblical characters in the fashions of their own times, certain traditions became fixed. A clean-shaven Hebrew prophet is almost unthinkable. (From: IBID)

The best known of all of the solar heroes is the biblical Samson, whose name could well have been derived from the Hebrew word shemesh, meaning Hair. Samson's courage and supernatural strength made him the champion of Israel against the Philistines, and his downfall came only when Delilah, bribed by the enemy, persuaded him to reveal the source of his great strength. He was finally seduced into telling her "if I be shaven, then my strength will go from me, and I shall become weak, and be like any other man." So while he slept upon her knees, Delilah had his seven locks shaven and magical power of hair. The origins of such strong convictions about the power of hair for good or evil are far more complex than the very obvious origins linking hair to sexual power and fertility.

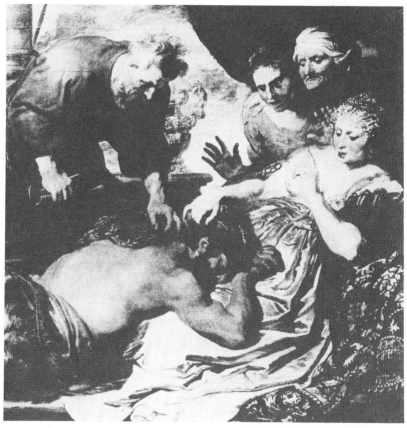

Figure 3. Samson and Delilah, by Dutch painter Anthony van Duck (1599-1641). In the biblical story the cutting off of Samson's hair deprived him of his strength – an example of a man's head hair 'displacing' his facial and body hair as a symbol of virility and power. (From: IBID)

Once Samson's strength had gone from him, the Philistines captured him with ease. Although they put out his eyes and bound him with fetters of brass, they did not allow for the fact that his hair would grow again, and as it did, his strength returned. He was able to tear down the pillars of the house to which his captors had brought him and he died along with his enemies in the ruins.

Although this is the best known story, the true original sun-hero is Gilgamesh. Although part of Babylonian legend, he is thought to have possibly been a real historical figure, a conqueror of the Euphrates Valley in the third millenium BC, who was later given the attributes of a solar deity. Sculptures depict him always with long, thick hair clustered into snaky twists, gripping a half-throttled lion under one arm. He was the prototype of both the Greek Hercules and the biblical Samson.

The Babylonians believed that after the seventh month of the year, the sun became enfeebled by a leprous disease that caused its hair to fall out. In the legend, therefore, Gilgamesh also grows sick at that time. Like the sun, he has to make a long journey over dark waters to purify himself so that 'the hair of his head is restored', and with it his power. Like the sun, he returns radiant and refreshed. The same idea pervades the saga of the Irish sun-hero Cuchulainn, who always falls ill on the eve of November as the dark season begins, and, to restore himself, sets out for the other world of Labraith's Isle.

Like Samson, Gilgamesh owed his misfortune to the seduction of a woman. In his case, Ishtar, whom he had slighted, afflicted him with a

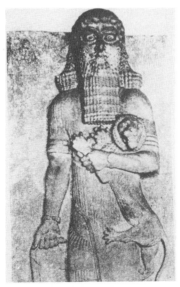

Figure 4. An 8th century BC bas-relief from Khorsabad of the Assyrian sun-hero Gilgamesh. The Gilgamesh legend has many points in common with that of the Greek Hercules, who also slew a lion with his bare hands and was also represented as a muscular, bearded figure. (From: IBID)

loathsome disease that caused his hair to fall out. Some may well see implications of venereal disease in these old legends, and it must be more than a coincidence that the Aztec word, nanahuatl, meaning 'afflicted with venereal disease' is also a name given to their sun-god. The sun-heroes were invariably sexual adventurers, and the age-old link between hair and virility is echoed in their conquests.

What man most admired in other men, he expected to find in his gods. Thus, he endowed his dieties with those human signs of strength and power, flowing locks and beards. In turn, the half-human, half-devine folk heroes who emerged in myth and legend inherited from both gods and men hair touched with divinity and possessed of magical power.

Primitive man's instinctive worship of the sun shows the link with hair very clearly. Here was a god who rose each day over the rim of the world to bring light and warmth and in some strange way nurtured life itself. And this god had hair which could be seen. The moment the shining face, too bright to gaze upon, slipped behind a cloud and again as it emerged, there were the separate rays of gleaming hair. Small wonder that the early Aryan settlers of India who worshipped the sun addressed their god as 'the long-haired' or 'the golden-haired', or that ancient hymns of the Hindu sacred book, the Rig-Veda, describe the solar god as 'the brilliant sun with flaming hair'. The same luxuriant locks adorned other sun-gods: the Greek Apollo, the Rhodian Helios, the Cunobelin of Gaul. While far away across the world, the Mexicans called their sun-god Quetzalcoatl, 'bushy haired' and the Aztecs of Central America named their god of the declining day Tzontemoc, 'of the abundant hair', indicating the long slanting rays of the evening sun. The Roman poet Claudian, living around AD 400. invoked their sun-god 'to scatter daylight abroad with more copious locks' and the ancient Egyptian's solar deity, Ra, was adorned 'with golden locks' from his head.

Of course, not only sun-gods were distinguished by long hair and beards to symbolize strength and power. Poseidon and Zeus in Greek mythology, Jupiter and Neptune in Roman, and Thor and Odin in Norse legends, were just a few of the hundreds of hairy powerful gods. Even Jehovah was traditionally represented with a beard.

Not surprisingly, superstitions and myths about hair were rife among humans and found expression not only in relatively harmless ways, such as Jews wearing beards or Frankish kings being forbidden from childhood to cut their hair, but also in more sinister ways. In particular, hair became associated with witchcraft and sorcery. Medicine men among the Haida Indians of British Columbia on one side of the Atlantic might neither cut nor comb their hair, nor might priests of many negro tribes, such as the Hos of West Africa on the other. Among the Masai in East Africa, not a single hair could be plucked from their beards without loss of magic power.

Across the world from east to west, the belief in a link between the hair and the soul left its mark on many cultures and played its part in magic and fear. North American Indians thought the hair imprisoned the soul, and that by scalping an enemy they captured the soul and prevented it from escaping and returning to seek revenge. Possession of the scalp also added to their own stock of magical power. The same basic idea in ancient Greece meant that until a lock of hair had been given to Prosperpina, the goddess of death, she would refuse to release the soul from the dying body.

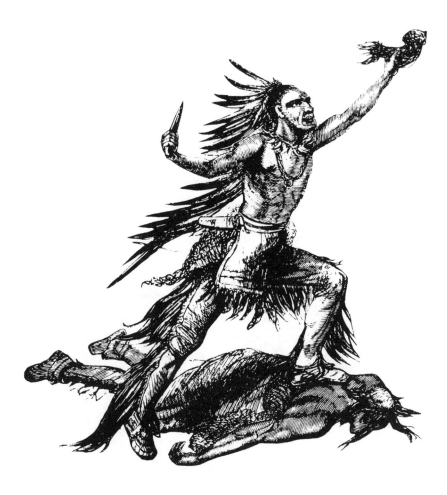

Figure 5.   Most American Indians learned the practice of scalping from white bounty hunters. Some tribes came to believe that scalping released the dead man's soul, but it also was a token taking of his manhood. (From: IBID)

Such widespread belief in the power of hair inevitably found its place in European witchcraft. Hair was considered so potent in Scotland that it was ominous even to meet a young woman with her head uncovered, and if a woman shook her hair at you, anything might happen. In 1633, Bessie Skebister was accused and convicted of causing disease in another woman, Margaret Mudie, whose cow had trespassed among Bessie's corn, simply by the deadly expedient of 'shaking of her hair'. When the climax of superstitious fear led in the end to the cruelties of witch hunts, it became common practice in Europe to shave the wretched suspects before handing them over to the torturers. According to Frazer, in his *Folk-lore in the Old Testament*, it was customary in France to shave the witch's whole body, partly to search for hidden marks of Satanic allegience and partly to deprive her of the strength and protection she derived from her hair. In 15th century Germany, inquisitor Cumanus shaved the whole bodies of 41 women before consigning them all to the flames.

Such excesses were not confined to Europe. A British writer, W. Crooke, in his book *The Folklore of Northern India*, published in 1896, describes how in the Province of Bastar 'if a man is adjudged guilty of witchcraft, he is beaten by the crowd, his hair is shaved, the hair being supposed to constitute his power of mischief. Women suspected of sorcery have to undergo the same ordeal.' Among the Bhils of central India, such hair from a witch was buried in the ground so 'that the last link between her and her former powers of mischief might be broken.' The Aztecs carried out a similar practice with the head of a witch cropped to remove supernatural forces.

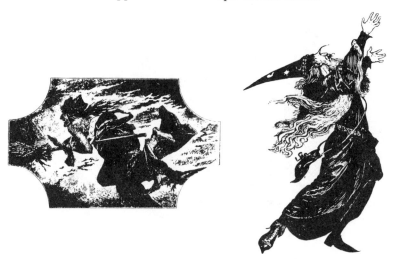

Figure 6. (a) Traditional white-bearded fair-tale wizard.
(b) The common conception of a witch – an ugly, hairy, skinny old bag on a broomstick. Her hairiness was the hairiness of evil, derived from her association with the hairy devil, and much of her power was believed to reside in her hair.

The human mind has always conceived of such forces working for good or evil, and just as hair was linked with divine power, usually benign, it was also linked with devils, demons, wizards and malevolent power, with hairiness a mark of bestiality. The devil's body is frequently depicted as hairy, along with horns and hooves, an inheritance perhaps from the goat-like Pan and satyrs of Greek mythology. Demons of the underworld are often shown covered with hair and Shakespeare even gave beards to his three weird sisters in Macbeth.

The association of evil spirits with beast-like qualities lies deeply buried in man's psyche. Traditionally, werewolves, vampires and other demon animals have been regarded as being in league with the devil. The wolf-man seems to be among the very oldest of mankind's dark dreads, linking Indian mythology with its rakshasas, mis-shapen giants with red hair and beards who devour human flesh, right down to the 17th century nursery story of Red Riding Hood. Wolf totems in the worship of dead ancestors saw the dead transformed perhaps into a divine type of superwolf.

Certainly, the werewolf myth was world wide. The Roman werewolf was commonly called a 'skin-changer' or 'turn-coat', and medieval legend followed up this idea, believing that while the werewolf kept his human form, his hair grew inward. When he wished to become a wolf, he simply turned himself inside out.

The Chinese, and later the Japanese, contented themselves with werefoxes, but in Europe wolfish gods were both feared and worshipped. The Germanic god Woden led his wild pack of wolves, as did the Thracian god, Zagreus, though he had a pack of maenads (raving women) clad in fox pelts.

The fear and fascination of werewolf legends dies hard. Outbreaks of a form of madness in which the raving patient believes himself a wolf, lycanthropy, have occurred, notably in France, even at the end of the 16th and 17th centuries, with gangs of rural poachers terrifying the countryside behind werewolf masks. The very name was nationally resurrected in Germany after World War I in the paramilitary Organization Werewolf, and as late as 1945, Himmler was calling upon his nation to harass 'like werewolves'.

Perhaps stories recounting the ravaging of Europe by the terrible beserkers and barbarian hordes, clad in animal pelts, passed by word of mouth down through the generations underlie these legends. But, it is possible it all goes further back to the time when shrinking forests drove our ancestors from the trees and forced fruit-eating creatures to evolve into remorseless killers, living on flesh. Stored in ancestral memory, the terrors and the traumas of those times could have emerged later in the werewolf myths and the terrible madness of lycanthropy, with its extraordinary compulsion to eat only raw and bloody meat. This change in habitat may underlie the very process which ended in man having 'unwanted hair'.

It is certainly a mystery why early man, like other primates, should have had so much hair but why modern man has come to have so little. While other

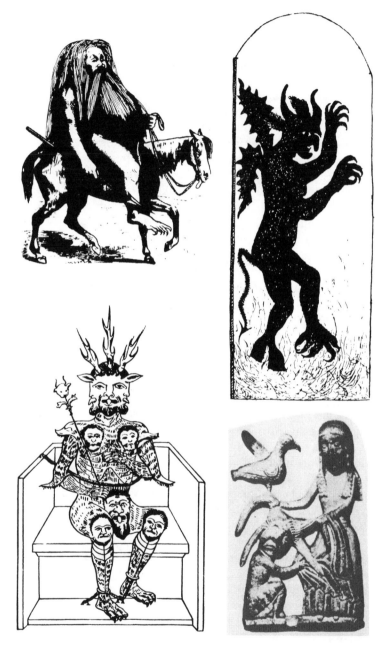

Figure 7. In most cultures the devil is depicted as hairy. The otherwise benign-looking devil on a horse (a) has a mane of hair to go with his clawed feet; the horned, winged devil (b) has a hairy tail; the seated devil (c) has no less than three beards. The Romanesque relief (d) shows a woman destroying a devil's power by plucking his head.

animals have retained fur and hair, why has the body hair of Homo sapiens become weaker, thinner, shorter and finer? It is easy to see that living in forests a good covering of body hair could protect against extremes of heat and cold, as well as against bumps, blows and abrasions. It could offer a handhold to enable the young to cling to the mother, provide padding against friction, and even offer a degree of camouflage. In contrast, living on the open plains, heavy hair covering would have been an embarrassment. As a hunter, competing with fierce nocturnal carnivores better equipped in tooth, claw and speed, man would sensibly choose to exert his lesser skills in daytime, despite the heat. Armed only with simple short-range weapons, he would need both to undertake long-sustained chases and to make quick rushes to catch and kill fast moving prey. By shedding his hairy impeding coat and increasing the number of sweat glands on his body surface, he would have been able to lose metabolic heat more quickly.

This was the theory which I found stood up best in my own book *Hair – Sex, Society and Symbolism* (Stein and Day, 1971). Probably many factors worked together. Evolution is not a planner but an opportunist, and exposed skin must have brought other advantages. It was less liable to offer a breeding ground for parasites, easier to keep clean and free of disease. It also afforded a clear identification and signaling device, particularly on the sexual level. Even among primates, males tend to be hairier than their female counterparts, and by extending this difference, the more naked human female could well have increased her sexual attraction. So, natural selection for all these reasons would tend to favor greater and greater hair loss, affecting the male also to a lesser degree.

No doubt naked skin might also add considerably to tactile sensation, heightening sexual excitement for mating couples. In his book *The Naked Ape,* zoologist Desmond Morris stresses the value of this to a species in which pair-bonding became important. Dr. Morris argues that the naked ape's survival depended on his success in transforming himself from a casual fruit-picking ape in the trees to an organized hunting ape on the plains, cooperating with other males. Such a degree of cooperation would only become possible if sexual rivalry was reduced to the minimum, and the unprotected females could be left safe from the advances of other males. So, this could, rather sadly, be the totally unromantic origin of the human need to fall in love, develop a pair-bond and remain (at least for the most part) faithful.

If we accept this theory, we still need to explain those special areas where we have retained dense hair, where hair is not 'unwanted', except in certain cultures who choose to shave head hair for religious reasons or depilate body hair for sexual preference.

The need for head hair is fairly obvious. The head above all needs protection, and similarly brows and lashes protect vulnerable eyes, while hair across the open passages of nose and ears acts as sieves against insects, dust and irritants in general.

But pubic and axillary hair present us with a different problem. Why did they remain? Both may serve as padding against friction, but as they do not appear until puberty, they seem to have survived as clear signals of sexual maturity. They almost certainly fulfill other sexual functions. Both the pubic and axillary hair grows in areas where the skin contains scent glands, whose secretions require exposure to air to develop their full odor. The tufts of hair thus release a distinctive scent that serves, or at least served primeval man, as a recognition signal and a stimulant to sexual play and mating.

All this is based only on intelligent guesswork about the past and on limited observation in the present. Even today, pubic hair is a sexual cynosure, and so desirable in most cultures that pubic wigs can be obtained.

Male hair, particularly facial hair, may also echo the value of epigamic hair, related to sexual dominance. Adult male monkeys have extra hair growth to form beards, moustaches and manes, all of which they use to give themselves a fierce appearance in threat displays and scuffles for power. There may well have been a time when human male hair had a similar epigamic function and so had a selective advantage in evolution. Charles Darwin believed that natural selection favored not only epigamic hair in the male, but also contrasting nakedness in the female. He believed our ancestors liked a woman with a fine head of hair but a naked body, except for those essentially sexual areas. Because body fur had no functional use to make its retention necessary, this nakedness became assimilated to the male, who retained only his vital epigamic hair.

Modern man is not, it seems, very different. In a special survey done for my book (*Hair – Sex, Society, Symbolism*) two-thirds of the women questioned were attracted by male body hair, and 80% of them were convinced that their own pubic hair was a weapon in their sexual armory. This was certainly confirmed by the men questioned, many of whom found it to be so strong a stimulant that it lead to instant erection.

However, such matters are often a matter of fashion or of cultural conditioning. Sometimes, even just a matter of personal preference. Even in the small sample our survey covered, we found four men who insisted on their partners removing pubic hair, while three-quarters of the men in this British survey preferred their partners remove axillary hair.

In general in our Western cultures, there is no record of men in general ever finding pubic hair 'unwanted'. Perhaps Shakespeare made the charms of woman's body hair most delightfully clear. While the ancient Egyptians and Greeks made depilation the rule for women, Shakespeare found it neither ugly nor unhygienic and maybe he should have the last words on the subject:

"Fondling she saith, 'since I have hemm'd thee here,
Within the circuit of this ivory pale
I'll be a park, and thou shalt be my deer:
Graze on my lips: and if those hills be dry
Stray lower, where the pleasant fountains lie.

Within this limit is relief enough,
Sweet bottom-grass, and high delightful plain,
Round rising hillocks, brakes obscure and rough,
To shelter thee from tempest and from rain:
Then be my deer, since I am such a park:
No dog shall rouse thee, tho'a thousand bark."

Venus and Adonis – William Shakespeare

12
The Roots of Hair

Robert B. Greenblatt, M.D.
R. Don Gambrell, JR., M.D.

In every generation, the man with a luxuriant head of hair has been either an object of admiration or derision, depending upon the time, clime and mood of the people; but, in contrast, the bald-headed man has forever been the butt of humor. The crowning glory of many a woman has been long, flowing locks of thick, luxuriant head hair, often with bouncing curls to outline her beautiful face. Fear strikes her heart when some of this hair becomes excessive in comb or brush, even without any signs of thinning. Let bald patches appear and she will stop at nothing to find the source of the failing scalp, sparing no expense to restore its original thickness. But, when unwanted hair appears on the face or chin, this same woman will endure every pain for its removal, leaving no stone unturned in seeking a permanent cure. Failing medical correction of this abomination, she may turn to quackery, sparing no expense to get to the roots of her problem. After all, the bearded lady is no longer popular, even at the country fair freak show or at the circus.

Still, one cannot help but wonder about today's trend. Not so many years ago, only women went in for the whole salon treatment: $20.00 razor cuts, blow drying, sprays, gels, coloring and conditioners – the whole expensive, narcissistic bit. Men, who may have moaned about the wife's hairdresser bills, made do with a $2.00 trip to the neighbourhood barbershop, a far cry from today's 'unisex' salon where both sexes entrust their locks to a fashionable stylist to the tune of $30.00 or $40.00 (or more) per session. Does all this mean, as some psychologists imply, that we are indeed embarking on a unisex era, in which you won't know the boys from the girls, at least not by their hair? Or, is it simply another chapter in man's preoccupation with his hair? A recent comedy movie, "Mr. Mom", depicted some of the humorous

things that can happen when typical mother-father roles are reversed, where
the father stays home to care for the children and the domestic chores while
the mother does the breadwinning.

Through the centuries, long and luxuriant hair has held some strange
fascination for both men and women. In his phylogenetic development, man
emerged not only erect, but also void of much of the thick pelage covering the
other primates. But man alone can grow excessively long head hair, and this
has often been considered a symbol of strength and masculinity. Witness
Samson, the epitome of this mystique – the Nazarite who slew 500 Philistines
with the jawbone of an ass. But when the treacherous Delilah gave him the
most infamous haircut in history, Samson was reduced to a weak and helpless
shadow of a man, blinded and imprisoned by his enemies. Ah, but when his
hair grew again, Samson tasted revenge, however brief.

This is probably not the whole story. Perhaps the mental anguish Samson
suffered on learning that he, a Nazarite, had been shorn of his hair was great
enough sorrow to throw him into physical decline. Or, more likely, perhaps
his fate paralleled that of an older legendary tribal hero who lost his strength
when his woman castrated him during a deep sleep, and thus weakened, he
fell into enemy hands.

Of course, this association with hair and masculinity has no scientific basis;
in fact, it is the eunuch who keeps his hair. Unlike beards, axillary and pubic
growth, head hair is not primarily hormonally dependent, even though the
hairline and thickness may be modified by hormones. Nor can it be considered entirely genetic. But it is safe to say that baldness in men follows a
genetic pattern, tempered by individual hormonal milieu.

Men castrated in their youth usually do not become bald, even if they have
a familial history of baldness. Indeed, bald men have been known on occasion
to regrow their hair following castration – a rather drastic solution to falling
hair, you'll agree! Still, the eunuch has enjoyed a rather gentle place in history.
In Chaucer's Canterbury Tales, for example, we have the gentle Pardoner who
had come straight from the court at Rome. "The Pardoner had hair as yellow
as wax," Chaucer wrote, "his locks hung down . . . over his shoulders. No
beard did he have, nor would ever have . . ."

The balding Louis XIV hit on a simpler and more fashionable solution – the
decorative wig. A little later, when England's Charles II was exiled to France,
these wigs struck his fancy, and he brought the fashion back to England when
he was restored to the throne in 1660. The vogue spread throughout Europe,
where it became fashionable as the style of the affluent and a symbol of honor
and culture. The wig is still worn in the courts of England (who can forget
Charles Laughton as the barrister in Witness for the Prosecution?), and serves as
a reminder that justice and the integrity of the law are continual and unchang-
ing – at least in theory. Millions are spent each year by countless men and
women on toupees and wigs, designed to resemble their former luxuriant or
fantasy hair. Hair transplants are also coming into vogue to hide baldness and

produce the appearance that used to be – or should have been. Funds are expended for hair restorers and often wasted on quackery in the hope of providing that image of what one's self should be.

On the other hand, the macho image, as portrayed by Yul Bryner or Telly Savalas, may be punctuated by artificial baldness – keeping the head completely shaven of all hair. Both men and women have long equated baldness or balding with virility; perhaps rightfully so, since male-pattern genetic baldness does not develop in the absence of testosterone. In contrast, Mahatma Gandhi also shaved his head, as do the Buddhist monks, yet he personally was known as a most gentle man, and one of the early perpetuators of non-violent protest action.

Sociologists and psychologists have had a field day with the more current symbolism attached to hair, especially the long-haired male spawned by the Beatles in the 1960s. Of course, history is full of long-haired rebels and original thinkers.

Jesus is pictured with long, flowing head hair and a full beard, which seems to have been recently confirmed by all the interest in the Shroud of Turin. Although he did not proclaim himself to be a revolutionary, his words and deeds convey that he was, in the best sense of the word. No other man has made such an impact or change in the course of history as Jesus of Nazareth. Flavius Josephus, the great first century Jewish historian, who chronicled the wars between the Jews and Rome, is portrayed with long hair, as was Muhammed (7th century), Moses Maimonides (12th century), Martin Luther (16th century), Victor Hugo (18th century), Walt Whitman (19th century), and Albert Einstein (20th century). Poets and painters, statesmen and politicians often distinguished themselves by their hair styles – from George Washington to John F. Kennedy, Disraeli to Lloyd George, Mozart to Stravinsky, Milton to Hemingway, to mention but a few.

In our day, long hair and beards have been the hallmark of the beatnik, the hippie, the disenchanted, the individualist. Hair length and style quickly reflect the mood of the day. For a while, it symbolized dissent, defiance, dissatisfaction with the status quo. For many, it became the badge proclaiming abhorrence of war in general and the Vietnam war in particular. But at times, the symbols get a bit mixed up. Some of our most fervent antiwar protests were directed at Lyndon Johnson, with the long hairs lined up on the side of peace and the short hairs on the side of war. It was also young against old, sexually liberated versus the traditionalists. But the images can change as quickly as hair grows, and before his death, President Johnson sported an over-the-collar mane of silver hair, and in retrospect of Watergate, some of his harshest critics are calling his presidency "the good old days . . ." And now, the more recent pictures of ex-Nixon aide H.R. Haldeman show even he is letting his hair grow, while reports from some campuses proclaim that short hair is the 'in' wave. The 1984 Democratic Presidential nominee, Walter Mondale, sports the more 'respectable' short hair, while his two closest but defeated rivals had moderately longer hair. Only the historians and pollsters can determine if there was an anti-hair protest vote that year.

And, too, the protesting beards of the sixties and seventies have become more respectable in the eighties. Several prominent and world-renowned endocrinologists hide their chins with full beards, as does the Surgeon General in the conservative Reagan administration. Doctors, lawyers, ministers, corporate executives, as well as singers and entertainers have brought respectability to facial hair.

What does all this prove? For one thing, it shows that there is nothing new in this obsession with hair. But if history has any lesson for the present, we may rest assured that whatever today's fad, chic or symbol, it too will undoubtedly pass.[1]

1. Greenblatt, R. B., The roots of hair. Medical Opinion, Sept. 1974

Jesus

Samson

Martin Luther

Charles II

Louis XIII

Washington

Victor Hugo

Mozart

Walt Whitman

Albert Einstein

13
Epilogue

Robert B. Greenblatt, M.D.
R. Don Gambrell, Jr., M.D.

WHAT OF THE FUTURE?

We cannot look ahead unless we look back at the past. For many years, the problem of unwanted hair was either ignored or treated with many modalities – some more effective than others. Plucking of hair is as old as civilization, and use of depilatories ranges from elephant dung, herbs and vegetable extracts, to chemical agents. Wax and honey preparations have been employed from time immemorial, and shaving has been used when other methods have failed. Thermolytic machines – some far more efficient than others – came into vogue only in the past 10 to 20 years.

What improvements in this field of endeavor may we expect in the future? No doubt, there will be better and more effective mechanical methods of hair removal – improved machines that will destroy the hair roots, painlessly and totally, utilized by technicians trained in the art. Electrolysis, as discussed in Chapter 1, is the principal method of hair destruction used today. It can be somewhat painful and at times can leave some scarring. Perhaps laser beams can be so pinpointed to ablate the hair root in a painless and nondisfiguring way. Improved technology should be able to use electric currents more efficiently and without any discomfort or scarring. Chemical depilatories should be perfected much like modern farming techniques, where products like Roundup (isopropylamine salt of glyphosate) can destroy weeds without adversely affecting the crops that are actively growing. Roundup is a foliage spray herbicide thought to be completely safe, certainly with nowhere near the toxicity of Paraquat or Agent Orange. Space-age computer technology should refine and improve current methods of unwanted hair removal and develop more desirable methods.

Hormonal methods of suppressing excessive androgens and proper more wide-spread use by physicians of preparations such as estrogens are discussed in Chapter 10. Estrogens will bind testosterone, decreasing the amount of free testosterone which stimulate the pilosebaceous apparatus. One way of hastening the future is patient education so they will seek medical aid at the onset of hirsutism. Today, it is much easier to prevent hirsutism and arrest its progression, than to remove the unwanted hair once it is established. If women will seek and the physician finds the source of abnormal hair stimulation in the early stages, modern endocrinology has the technical knowledge to prevent the continued accumulation of unwanted hair. No doubt the future will bring improved diagnostic techniques and hormonal therapeutic modalities.

The future of hormonal manipulation could also be hastened toward the present if antihirsute preparations, in use in Europe for more than a decade, were made available in the United States. Cyproterone and cyproterone acetate (fully discussed in Chapter 10) have strong anti-androgenic and progestational activity (progesterone is the hormone of pregnancy and the one produced the last half of the menstrual cycle that keeps periods regular). Improvement in both acne and hirsutism after treatment with cyproterone acetate has been widely demonstrated overseas; however, the Food and Drug Administration has not yet approved its usage in the United States.

When cyproterone was combined with ethinyl estradiol for ovarian suppression, improvement in acne and seborrhea was reported in all patients and hirsutism decreased in 60% to 80%. The side effects were those of some of the original high dosage oral contraceptives, along with tiredness, lassitude, and loss of libido. Also, as discussed in Chapter 10, moderate to high dosage oral contraceptives used until the mid-1970s are effective in themselves in treating and suppressing the progression of hirsutism. Whether the low dosage birth control pills most often prescribed today, especially the ultra low dosage pills of the future, will be as effective in reversing hirsutism, remains to be proven.

The introduction of an effective and safe antiandrogen into our therapeutic armamentarium has been a goal long sought. Long-term adrenal and ovarian suppression have undesirable side effects and interfere with the organs' normal hormonal function during treatment and during the extended period of recovery after discontinuation of therapy. A suitable antiandrogen is highly desirable for the management of hirsutism. Ideally, such a compound should be devoid of all other hormonal activity and should be rapidly cleared from the body.

Clinical and animal studies were undertaken by Greenblatt and Mahesh several years ago with a promising antiandrogen, 17α-methyl-β-nortestosterone (Fig. 1).[1,2] However, the expense of manufacturing this agent and stringent requirements of the Food and Drug Administration for further safety testing resulted in loss of interest by the manufacturers in promoting this agent. In the preliminary studies of this compound at the Medical College

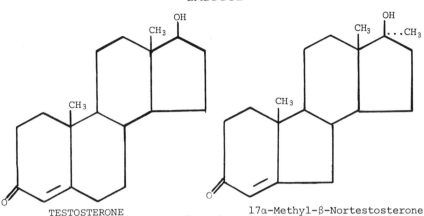

TESTOSTERONE
17α-Methyl-β-Nortestosterone

Figure 1.

of Georgia, 55 patients with varying combinations of acne and hirsutism were studied before 17α-methyl-β-nortestosterone was withdrawn from clinical testing. Although the criterion of improvement was based on subjective judgement, nonetheless, the results were quite obvious. Beneficial results were observed in 26 or 35 patients with acne (74.3%). Lessening of hirsutism was noted in 21 of the 40 patients studied (52.5%). The best effects were achieved with dosages ranging from 200 to 400 mg per day. Improvement in acne frequently was noted within a short time of one or more weeks. The more severe cases of acne showed the greatest improvement, while the diminution of hirsutism was more gradual and not related to the degree of hypertrichosis. On discontinuation of therapy, acne recurred in all patients, and 62% of the patients reported further progression of hirsutism.

The only side effect reported was gynecomastia (enlargement of the breasts) in two males treated for acne over prolonged periods. Other than this, the relative absence of untoward reactions and the lack of derangement in the other hormone-secreting glands were features of this drug.

The best and most rational management of the manifestations of increased sensitivity to endogenous androgens is through the administration of an antiandrogen. The excellent results obtained years ago, although temporary, offer promise to the long-term approach in the treatment of acne and idiopathic hirsutism. It is hoped that continued search for the ideal antiandrogen will continue.

The future should bring better agents which either interfere with steroid hormone synthesis or block the active androgen metabolites that stimulate the pilosebaceous apparatus. As discussed in Chapter 10, a major breakthrough in this direction came two or three years ago with the discovery that an ulcer medicine, Tagamet (cimetidine), a histamine blocker, would make unwanted hair go away in some women. This apparently works by blocking the final steps of androgen stimulation at the level of the hair follicle, the conversion of testosterone to dihydrotestosterone (DHT), which is the most stimulating of all the androgens. Unfortunately, Tagamet not only is an expensive drug, it is only effective in decreasing hirsutism in less than 50% of afflicted patients. Slightly more effective and less expensive is the anti-aldosterone drug spironolactone, which also interferes with testosterone production with only a few and rather insignificant side effects. Other agents will no doubt come to the fore that will prove helpful in the further management of hirsutism.

Finally, the mutual cooperation of physician and electrologist is essential for the betterment of the patient suffering from the curse of unwanted hair, whether it be hereditary or due to a glandular disorder. Electrologists should find physicians with the expertise to diagnose and effectively arrest the progression of hirsutism for referral of their patients having hair removed. Physicians should also provide their patients with a list of competent electrologists, for referral of their patients once the hormonal cause of hirsutism has been established and an effective therapeutic program implemented. It is an exercise in futility to continually electrolyze hair in the presence of excess androgens, thereby promoting ever increasing hirsutism. Once the progression of the hirsutism has been slowed to a standstill, then and only then can electrolysis be utilized with the most efficiency. Perhaps even other methods that are not thought of today will be developed in the future for the simplest and most effective control of unwanted hair.

References

1. Zarate, A., Mahesh, V. B., Greenblatt, R. B., Effect of an antiandrogen, 17α-methyl-β-nortestosterone, on acne and hirsutism. J Clin Endocrinol Metab 26:1394, 1966
2. Dalla Pria, S., Greenblatt, R. B. and Mahesh, V. B., An antiandrogen in acne and idiopathic hirsutism. J Invest Derm 52:348, 1969

Index